Death in Zion National Park

Stories of Accidents and Foolhardiness in Utah's Grand Circle

Randi Minetor

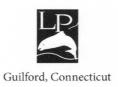

Guilford, Connecticut

An imprint of Globe Pequot

Distributed by NATIONAL BOOK NETWORK

British Library Cataloguing in Publication Information Available

Library of Congress Cataloging-in-Publication Data Available

ISBN 978-1-4930-2893-1 (paperback)
ISBN 978-1-4930-2894-8 (e-book)

♾™ The paper used in this publication meets the minimum requirements of American National Standard for Information Sciences—Permanence of Paper for Printed Library Materials, ANSI/NISO Z39.48-1992.

Printed in the United States of America

CONTENTS

Preface iv

Introduction: The Perils of the Vertical Vacation vi

CHAPTER 1. Trapped in an Instant:
Flash Floods in the Narrows 1

CHAPTER 2. Rising Waters:
Incidents in Other Canyons 24

CHAPTER 3. Crossing the Neck: Angels Landing............ 48

CHAPTER 4. The Edge of Forever:
Falls from High Places 69

CHAPTER 5. Daring Fate: Climbing, Canyoneering,
and BASE Jumping Accidents 90

CHAPTER 6. Sudden Darkness:
The Zion–Mt. Carmel Tunnel 122

CHAPTER 7. Due Process: Deaths by Suspicious
Circumstances.. 132

CHAPTER 8. On the Road: Vehicular Deaths................. 144

CHAPTER 9. Unclassified: Deaths by
Unusual Causes.. 151

Epilogue: How to Stay Alive in Zion National Park..... 164

Appendix: List of Deaths 1908–2016 in
Chronological Order 175

Bibliography 179

Index.. 199

About the Author... 208

PREFACE

This book details the ninety-two deaths that have taken place in Zion National Park, as well as some near-death experiences included to illustrate the kinds of hazards this park presents to the adventurous visitor. Most of these incidents have taken place since the park achieved federal protection as Mukuntuweap National Monument in 1909, and as Zion National Park in 1919. This is not surprising, as the park's popularity has increased steadily since that time to record attendance of 4,317,028 in 2016.

There may actually be more than ninety-two people whose deaths took place in the park, but the media and other sources do not always make note of people who happened to die of natural causes during their visit. If it appears I have missed the passing of your loved one, please feel free to get in touch with me at author@minetor.com to provide any factual information you may have available. I will be sure to include it in the book's next edition.

As you read this book, please keep in mind that while more and more people visit Zion every year, on average only one to two people per year actually perish while at the park. The news in recent years included one incident in 2015 that took the lives of seven people, and pairs of climbers or hikers sometimes meet death at the same time, but the overall number of fatal incidents remains low. Please do not take this collection of stories as any indication that you should not visit this extraordinary park. See these instead as opportunities for you to learn the best and most effective skills for approaching any trail, rock face, river, road, or tunnel in Zion—and in any other wilderness area. *Death in Zion National Park* should serve as reinforcement of the basic rules of safety recommended to every visitor by the National Park Service. (I've collected these guidelines and survival tips and included them in the epilogue of this book.)

Zion National Park is my favorite of all the national parks—and as of this writing, I have visited 306 of the 417 units of the National Park Service, so I have some significant basis for comparison. I urge you to visit this park, explore its winding trails, discover its hanging gardens and slot canyons, ride the scenic roads in a car or on a bicycle, and gaze at the magnificent views of stratified red sandstone towering two thousand feet above the canyon floor. You will see no landscape on earth to rival this one, so make the most of your visit by venturing into its concealed areas, from the splendor of Refrigerator Canyon to the power of the eighty-foot waterfall at Upper Emerald Pool. Any wilderness area presents some risks, but when you take a few simple safety precautions and heed the advice of the park's rangers, your visit will be filled with wonders beyond your imagination.

INTRODUCTION: THE PERILS OF THE VERTICAL VACATION

You are about to read of the ninety-two people who arrived at Zion National Park expecting to have the time of their lives but all ended up dead. There is no kinder way to put this, so I want to be as upfront as possible with you about the contents of this book. It's the result of significant research: an extensive review of media coverage, official documents, and other forms of investigation, and my own efforts to discern the facts in each case based on the information available.

All of the stories you are about to read are true, to the best of my ability to determine the truth. In many cases I attempted to retrieve records of police and FBI investigations, using the Freedom of Information Act and Utah's Government Records Access and Management Act (GRAMA) to request aged files. I discovered that Washington County Sheriff's Office records dating back before 1997 are not available, making it quite impossible to determine what conclusions might have been drawn in older cases. Even the FBI did not have records of continuing investigations in deaths that were deemed to have occurred under suspicious circumstances, leaving us with no further clues once the media coverage ran its course. I am sorry to leave my readers with loose ends, but facts are facts, and not all cases could be solved.

Death in Zion National Park also reveals the tremendous search and rescue operations available to the people who visit here—the professionals, volunteers, and regional resources that penetrate the park's most treacherous landscapes to rescue people when they can, and when this is not possible, to bring out the remains of someone's loved one and allow the family to achieve closure. I wish I could detail for you the thousands of successful rescues the area's search teams complete: the retrieval of hundreds of people every year who stray off of trails, become lost or injured, or realize in a moment of sudden clarity that they have truly taken on more than they can handle. These visitors come home safely each season thanks to the tireless efforts of these heroes; only a tiny fraction—usually fewer than two people per year—lose their lives.

You will find that I have treated these incidents with respect, as I must consider the number of times I myself could have made a wrong turn in the wilderness and ended up just like the people who did not come home. While some of these stories might encourage a snicker behind closed doors and a sense of schadenfreude—a superiority to those who wandered off into a slot canyon, for example, and were met with a sixty-foot wall of waterborne debris—most of these accidents and incidents could happen to any of us. Most important, every tale has something to teach us.

The vast majority of these stories illustrate the results of uncommon bad luck: a rock that turned underfoot, a change in the weather just minutes after a party left cellular phone range, a knot not tied at the end of a rope, or a patch of ice in the worst possible place. A few happened because of neglect or foolishness, and a number of incidents took place for the sheer cussedness of attempting them—a grit and determination that turned out to be misguided. Perhaps worst of all, a handful were deliberate acts of desperation: three suicides, a fall that led to a murder trial, an unsolved case involving a pool of blood and a bloody backpack, and one death at the end of a night of drunkenness.

If this book encourages you to go to Zion National Park for no other reason than to see the peak of Angels Landing, the windings of the Narrows, the waterfalls of Emerald Pools, the mile-long darkness of Zion–Mt. Carmel Tunnel, and the depths of Kolob, Keyhole, and Pine Creek Canyons, then I will consider my efforts here a rousing success. Go, if you must, to see where people met bad ends, but stay to savor the views of vermillion cliffs, variegated rock faces, sparkling waters, and parti-colored sunsets. Zion is my favorite of all of America's national parks, and I am delighted to have this opportunity to invite you to see it for yourself.

Be careful out there.

CHAPTER 1

Trapped in an Instant: Flash Floods in the Narrows

THE NAMES OF THE FOURTEEN HIKERS IN THE NARROWS OF Zion Canyon on July 27, 1998, did not become part of the record reported in the *Salt Lake Tribune* two days later, but their gruesome find certainly did—and the report, at least in the short term, chilled many a hiker's enthusiasm for braving the waters of the North Fork of the Virgin River.

The Virgin River sculpts a dramatic and compelling corridor through the heart of Zion National Park, one that lures otherwise cautious hikers to take on a challenge entirely different from the ones they find on dry land. Here sandstone walls stretch upward for a thousand feet or more, allowing a glistening ribbon of water to find its way between them with only twenty or thirty feet of tolerance on either side. Sunlight generally forsakes this slim waterway, making this a dim or even murky journey—but when a shaft of natural light casts a momentary glow on a towering wall, the effect can be so remarkable that hikers pause to admire the play of sun and shadow against the folds of sandstone glowing in shades of vermillion, white gold, and mahogany.

On the floor of the canyon, the Virgin River polishes the rocks in its bed into slippery spheres, making a hike through even ankle-deep water tricky at best. The effect is like walking on "buttered bowling balls," as my husband phrased it during our most recent hike through the canyon. Every hiker knows—or discovers, much to his or her chagrin—that a sturdy walking stick is an absolute must, providing a necessary third point of contact with the ground while the hiker feels for a stable foothold with each cautious step forward. In Springdale, the park's entrance town, a viable industry has developed to provide Narrows hikers with canyoneering shoes, neoprene socks, walking sticks, dry suits in winter (when the water temperature drops to thirty-four degrees Fahrenheit), and wet suits in summer to help prevent soaking-wet hikers from developing hypothermia in the chilly shade of the upper canyon.

The bulk of the visitor traffic begins at the south end of the canyon where the park shuttle stops at the Temple of Sinawava, with hikers beginning their journey on the easy Riverside Walk. At the end of the mile-long paved path, it's time to plunge into the water and hike in the river to the canyon's narrowest point, about two and a half miles up the canyon. Here delighted visitors discover the slot canyons, gorgeous examples of the interplay of water, sandstone, and light as the walls stand barely twenty feet apart. "This is the slot canyon that all other slot canyons are compared to," writes photographer Joe Braun on his website, Joe's Guide to Zion National Park.

For casual hikers eager to see the best that Zion has to offer, this short but strenuous trek offers tremendous rewards in multiple megabytes of photos, access to hidden natural wonders that cannot be seen from any road, and bragging rights: Only the bravest visitors venture past the end of the Riverside Walk to see the magic in the heart of Zion Canyon.

Those who crave a more challenging experience of the canyon take the route less traveled, beginning at the north end at Chamberlain's Ranch. The daunting sixteen-mile route usually takes two days (though some power hikers finish it in one) and involves an overnight stay at one of the twelve designated campsites along the North Fork of the Virgin River. The park requires hiking parties to obtain a permit to hike the Narrows from the north end, and to make a reservation to use one of the campsites. This allows the park to control the number of people who hike the Narrows at any one time—but equally important, the permit and campsite reservation give the rangers a fairly good idea of where hikers are at any given time. If anything goes wrong and the hikers do not arrive safely at the end of the hike within a few hours of their expected time, search and rescue crews can deduce how far along the party might be.

Why the concern? While hiking the Narrows at its most shallow may result in an unplanned dunking into the water or, at worst, a twisted ankle, there's a greater danger from the middle of July to the end of August. Just as Zion's shuttle buses become jammed with passengers and the trails are crowded with day-trippers and visitors from around the world, torrential thunderstorms begin to pop up regularly in the mountains north of the park. Hikers in the Narrows report looking up past the canyon walls to see bright blue sky even as rain drenches the land twenty or thirty miles away. As the rain falls and the runoff from the desert and mountains swells the volume of the Virgin River, all that water flows into Zion Canyon.

Once inside, the volume of water becomes concentrated as it squeezes between the monolithic walls. The water level rises instantly, racing down the canyon at rates as high as four thousand cubic feet per second—and as the canyon becomes even narrower, the water level rises again. What may have begun as a few extra inches of water high in the mountains now speeds down the center of the canyon, reaching well over hikers' heads and creating a deadly situation for people who have been lulled into a sense of security by the patches of clear blue sky they see above them. If they are caught on low ground, they may be swept away by the current's force.

Because of Zion's unique topography, hikers also may find themselves without the ability to climb to safety. Flood-waters cover all the riverbed sandbars and scraps of land at the bottom of the canyon, and walls scoured by centuries of such floods offer no ledges or even footholds to help people climb to a higher point on the rock face. Hikers, climbers, and canyoneering enthusiasts, including some lifelong experts, have found themselves trapped on a point too low for safety. Others manage to scramble up to a point above the water, remaining stranded on a ledge until the water recedes. This can take many hours, an uncomfortable situation for hikers who thought they were on a day trip and who did not pack enough extra food, dry clothing, and water to last into another day.

So on Monday afternoon, July 27, 1998, when 0.47 inches of rain fell at Zion National Park headquarters and the Lava Point area west of the Narrows received 0.37 inches, parties of hikers—fourteen people in all—became trapped overnight about two miles upriver from the Temple of Sinawava parking area. They managed to scramble to higher ground as the water level rose three feet in a matter of minutes, and as the flow increased from 110 cubic feet to 740 cubic feet per second, making wading in the roiling river impossible. They made makeshift camps, getting as comfortable as they could while keeping a close eye on the current for any sign that the depth might become passable once again.

That's how the hikers spotted the body.

It floated by them at about 5:00 p.m., battered significantly by rocks it had encountered in the swift current. No medical expertise was required to determine that the person had most likely drowned in the flash flood.

Immediately seeing the need to retrieve this person's remains, several of the hikers worked together to reach the body, bring it to a patch of ground, and secure it there. It remained in place until early Tuesday morning, when the river had returned to a manageable level and the hikers could make their way out of the canyon. They reported their find to the first ranger they could locate.

When Zion's search and rescue squad entered the Narrows, it located the body where the hikers had secured it. Determining who the victim was, however, became a tricky process. "There was no identification on the man, and we haven't heard any reports about a missing person," park spokesman Denny Davies told the *Salt Lake Tribune*. The recovery team ventured an educated guess that the man was in his forties, and that he weighed between 230 and 250 pounds. Washington County sheriff Glenwood Humphries noted that the body had taken a severe beating in the swiftly flowing current, making it that much harder to achieve a solid identification. Whoever this person was, he had not obtained a permit from the park to hike the canyon, and he had not made an advance reservation for a campsite. His identity was a complete mystery.

On Tuesday evening, however, park investigators found an unlocked vehicle parked in Zion Canyon with two wallets in it, and they matched one of the driver's license photos with the unidentified body. They determined that the victim was twenty-seven-year-old Ramsey E. Algan of Long Beach, California. Two other hikers who had emerged from the canyon after the flash flood confirmed what seemed to be the case: Algan had been hiking with another man, and that man had not returned to his car either. Park search and rescue teams now had to face the fact that they had another hiker to find—and the chances were slim that they would find him alive.

On Wednesday, July 29, Acting Chief Ranger David Buccello coordinated the second search along the Virgin River, breaking the searchers into teams to explore five sectors of the park. He also engaged the assistance of Rocky Mountain Rescue Dogs from Salt Lake City. "The search dogs can be a great help in searching the debris piles left after such a flood," Buccello said in a statement released by the National Park Service. South of the park, Washington

County sheriff's deputy Kurt Wright led search efforts on the chance that the second man's body might have been carried downstream and beyond the park's boundaries on the strong storm current.

On Wednesday morning, July 30, searchers discovered the body of the second man about a mile and a half upstream from where Algan's body was first spotted. Paul Garcia, a thirty-one-year-old man from Paramount, California, was located in a debris pile where his body had snagged during the flash flood.

Park officials were quick to use this tragedy to reinforce the message that those planning to hike the Narrows need to check with park rangers at a visitor center or ranger station before venturing up or down the Virgin River. "We cannot stress too strongly that visitors need to heed these flash flood warnings and plan alternate trips that don't include slot canyons," acting park superintendent Eddie Lopez told the *Salt Lake Tribune*. He urged hikers to get updated weather information before venturing into any narrow or slot canyon, and to delay their hike if thunderstorms are predicted.

To Hike or Not to Hike

Park rangers at Zion move quickly to put a range of warnings in place when flash floods are possible in the Narrows. Hikers who apply for permits at ranger stations receive sincere and concerned discouragement from rangers if rainstorms are in the forecast, and signs are posted at the Narrows trailheads, warning hikers that flooding may be imminent. "Unfortunately, many people ignore the warnings and enter the Narrows," spokesperson Davies told the

Deseret News on the day Algan's body was retrieved. When asked if the victim should have known a flash flood warning was in effect, Davies responded simply: "Yes."

Why would anyone hike the Narrows when there's a flash flood in the forecast? For vacationers who have planned a hike up or down the Narrows as a central part of their Zion visit, timing can become a greater priority than the potential for danger. The special challenges of hiking, climbing, or canyoneering in the Narrows make it a bucket-list experience for many visitors—and after months or even years of planning, scrapping the hike because of rain may feel like the coward's way out.

The potential for life-threatening danger is very real, however. To date, fifteen people have perished in the Narrows when they were caught in flash floods, and many others have sustained injuries in their scramble to get out of the path of rushing water. There is no way to tally how many hikers have been forced to wait for hours or even overnight after they've succeeded in reaching higher ground—and untold numbers of these hikers made plans only for a day hike or for a single night in camp, finding themselves without sufficient food, water, warm clothing, or dry items to make their unscheduled extra time in the Narrows as bearable as possible.

With the wealth of information outlets available today, it's easy for would-be Narrows hikers to get the weather updates they need to determine if they should postpone their excursion for a day or two to avoid flash flood activity. The Zion National Park website's Current Conditions page, at www.nps.gov/zion/planyourvisit/conditions.htm, provides a number of links to water level information and flash flood forecasts, including the National Weather Service Forecast Office's page on all of southern Utah's parks: www.wrh.noaa .gov/slc/flashflood. There's even a link to the US Geological Survey's flow rate data for the Virgin River, so serious water information enthusiasts can delve into the trends in cubic feet per second. For people who just want to check the forecast, links to the National Weather Service (weather.gov) provide radar maps and the percentage chance of rain.

Descriptions of the Narrows hikes found on the park's website (www.nps.gov/zion/planyourvisit/thenarrows.htm) make it clear that this is not a hike for the timid. "Hiking the Zion Narrows means hiking in the Virgin River," the website explains. "At least 60% of the hike is spent wading, walking, and sometimes swimming in the stream. There is no maintained trail; the route is the river. The current is swift, the water is cold, and the rocks underfoot are slippery. Flash flooding and hypothermia are constant dangers. Good planning, proper equipment, and sound judgment are essential for a safe and successful trip."

There is no way to judge how many people's lives have been saved by the availability of data, the emphatic warning signs, and the advice of rangers in the park; we rarely hear about people who are dissuaded from making a dangerous hike into the wilderness. We do know, however, that while people find themselves trapped by a flash flood in the Narrows every year, only a handful of these floods have led to hikers' deaths. The most significant of these include the flash flood of 1961, one other deadly incident in 2015 in Keyhole Canyon, and a highly controversial flood in Kolob Canyon that took the lives of two adults and endangered a third adult and five children.

THE FLASH FLOOD OF 1961

"If Linda hadn't heard the roar," John Dearden of Park City, Utah, told the Provo *Daily Herald*, "nobody would have been alive."

Some describe the summer storms in southwest Utah as monsoons, sudden bursts of hard, pelting rain that flood dry creek beds until roads and bridges disappear under the flow. On Sunday, September 17, 1961, a cloudburst followed by steady rain dumped a whopping 0.79 inches of rain on parts of Utah, saturating the ground in advance of the more powerful storm to come. Monday's rain inundated Zion National Park and the surrounding area with an additional 1.33 inches, washing out the main bridge at the park's south entrance near Springdale and closing Highway 15 from St. George. Water engorged the Virgin River as the rain sluiced over the sandy soil and spilled down the riverbanks. As the rain continued to fall, the river swelled and gathered speed— and the force of it rushed into the Narrows.

Inside the canyon on Sunday morning, twenty-six hikers on a tour conducted by SOCOTWA Expeditions were well along an eighteen-mile hike they had begun on Saturday morning. Expecting clear weather—as reported by the local weather service when group leaders checked on Saturday morning—they had arrived by bus from Salt Lake City and entered the canyon from the Navajo Lake area in Dixie National Forest, heading south along the North Fork of the river. Nineteen teens and seven adults made their way along the spectacular slot canyons, keeping an unhurried pace between the two-thousand-foot-high canyon walls. They camped in the Narrows on Saturday night and continued on Sunday morning, entering an area well known for having no alternate routes and few opportunities to reach high ground.

They reached the confluence of Kolob Creek with the Virgin River at about noon on Sunday, and leader Robert Perry, an Air National Guardsman, led nine of the hikers on a side trip into Orderville Canyon. That's when Linda McIntyre let out a yell, and Perry heard the flood coming toward them. "The first indication of trouble was a thunderlike noise he heard in back of the group," the *Salt Lake Tribune* reported. When he turned around, Perry saw "a wall of muddy water, bristling with driftwood, tree trunks and limbs."

Perry decided that they should turn back. "We got to the mouth of the canyon and found Carla Larson standing knee deep in water," he told the *Tribune*. The girl was stranded on a high spot in the river, with deep water all around her. "We had to swim about ten yards to get to her. Someone asked, 'what next.'" Several group members provided their backpacks as flotation devices, and they towed Carla to higher ground and comparative safety.

"We knew a terrific flood had come down through the canyon," said Perry, "but we didn't realize how bad it was." Inexplicably, the weather was still clear. Half an hour would pass before the rain arrived in the Narrows—and then "you couldn't see a hundred yards across the gulch," he said. "I've been in hurricanes before, but they couldn't hold a candle to this storm."

Perry led his party up Orderville Canyon and found high ground, where they made a shelter from their ponchos and "huddled together in wet sleeping bags for warmth."

They passed a terrifying night in Orderville Canyon, with no idea how the other sixteen people in their tour were faring in the storm and flood.

"The rain-swollen stream suddenly grew to a 14-foot crest," the *Daily Herald* reported, "and bore down on them in a canyon only 12 feet wide in places."

Luckily, the group had reached an area of the Narrows where the walls provided some hand- and footholds, as well as ledges where they could escape the massive torrent of river water. Perched on sandbars and shelves of rock with the river rushing just below them, the members of the party could not see who had found their way up the canyon walls and who may have been swept away by the raging water. They remained pinned down throughout the night, hopeful that all of their friends and guides had scrambled to safety.

"The water came up to within a foot of us—we couldn't have gone any further, the rock wall was straight up," said Dearden.

Hiker Lyle Moss told the *Salt Lake Tribune* that he and two other hikers managed to climb up on top of a sandbar, but the water came to within six inches of where they were standing.

"Long time residents of the area say it was the heaviest rainstorm to hit the Zion Park area in nearly 25 years," the *Tribune* reported. "Rain gauges at park headquarters caught one and 43 hundredths inches of precipitation during the storm."

Twenty-two hours passed before the water had finally receded enough for the hikers to make their way out. On the ground at last, they found the riverbed muddier than when they began and loaded with debris—fallen branches, twigs, and dirt that formed irregular dams and obstacles to their progress. The ten who had passed the night in Orderville Canyon met up with nine other members of the party about a mile and a half downstream, and they began to hear the fate of some of the others. One group of boys and girls had found safety on the opposite side of the canyon from Lyle Moss, and they watched in horror as forty-eight-year-old Walter Scott, the leader of the group, and two younger boys drifted by in a current moving at an estimated twenty-five miles per hour.

When nineteen of the original twenty-six hikers emerged from the Narrows at the Riverside Walk on Monday afternoon, they found that search and rescue crews were already looking for them. Tour bus driver Dave Randall had arrived at the Temple of Sinawava on Sunday afternoon to pick up the hikers and take them home to Salt Lake—and when the tour group did not arrive, Randall moved quickly to notify park officials.

The hikers also learned that two of their comrades had already been pulled from the river. Young Vance Justett, a thirteen-year-old Springdale resident, discovered Walter Scott's body in Springdale on Monday when the boy went to the river to see how much damage the flood had done. He told Washington County deputy sheriff Dick Barnes that he saw a pair of legs in a pile of driftwood that the water had swept onto the shore. "So swift was the torrent that Mr. Scott's clothes were ripped off and only a pair of white tennis shoes remained on the body," the *Tribune* reported. "The victim's body was swept almost ten miles from where the party was struck by the torrent, near the junction of Kolob Creek and the Virgin River." Perry told the *Salt Lake Tribune* that Scott had brought up the rear of the expedition to remain with some of the boys in the party who had trouble organizing their equipment after their night of camping.

Not far from the spot where Scott was found, the body of thirteen-year-old Steve Florence, a junior high school student from Park City, was discovered lodged in a pile of driftwood, about 4:00 p.m. on Monday. The remains of seventeen-year-old Ray Nichols came to light at about 2:00 p.m. Monday, lodged between two trees near the park's South Campground. Nichols was a student at East High School in Salt Lake City.

When the exhausted hikers arrived on Monday with four of their comrades still not in evidence, a search began for Alvin Nelson, Frank Johnson, Kenneth Webb, and Doug Childs. Waiting families and searchers were overjoyed when fifty-year-old Webb and Childs, a boy of thirteen, sloshed their way out of the Virgin River and turned up at the park headquarters at about 5:00 p.m., both alive and well. They had climbed onto an embankment to take a picture when they saw the flood coming at them, but they could not communicate with the people ahead of them. They stayed on the high ground as the flood overtook their position, watching the water come up all the way to their knees before it began to subside. Webb decided to wait until they were sure the entire storm was over before making their way out of the canyon.

The ordeal was not quite over for Doug Childs, however. It fell to him to identify the body of his friend Steve Florence. "The Childs youth looked at the human wreckage of what was once his friend, [and] whispered almost inaudibly, 'that's Steve,'" the *Tribune* said.

The twenty-one survivors of the flash flood of 1961 were Albert Anderson, John Bangerter, Doug Childs, Bonnie Darger, John and Allen Dearden, Lila Fieden, Katherine Grim, Carol Harmon, Thomas Katwok, Carla Larson, Linda and Margaret McIntyre, Thad Merriman, Lyle Moss, Robert Perry, Adene Scott, Thomas Spencer, Leif Spondeck, Tommy Terry, and Kenneth Webb.

By Monday night there was still no sign of Nelson or Johnson. The park service sent a search party into the Narrows on Tuesday morning in hopes of finding the two young men alive, while jeep posses from Washington and Iron Counties searched along the Virgin River from the southern park boundary all the way to St. George.

The searchers soon discovered that the volume of water that had passed through the canyon brought with it massive quantities of silt, sand, rock, and other debris, a load as dangerous as the water itself. As the search wore on through the day Tuesday and broadened to include forty miles along the length of the Virgin River, the rescue teams surmised that the two missing seventeen-year-old Salt Lake City boys were buried under layers of newly arrived gravel and sand. The parents of the boys waited in the park as ground and air crews scoured the area for any clue that could lead searchers to the bodies. Cleanup crews, usually assigned to clearing driftwood and moving sand to restore the river's normal flow, had the grisly task of continuing the search as well.

Equally challenging, the river had not yet returned to its normally shallow level, making it difficult and even dangerous for the search to continue in some parts of the canyon. Sheriff Ray Renouf of Washington County finally called off the search Tuesday evening, promising the families of the two missing boys that the effort would continue at an intensive level once the waters had receded enough to allow crews to see the bottom of the river.

With less water and more debris visible over the next several days, searchers continued to try to locate the missing boys. "Searchers scoured a mile and a half stretch of the Virgin River from the southern edge of Zion Park through Springdale Thursday, but found no trace of the missing youths," the *Daily Herald* reported. The hunt beyond the Narrows continued on the theory that the boys' bodies may have been carried out of the park on the river's storm surge. The Washington County sheriff's department spent Friday, September 22, searching eight miles of the river with six hunting dogs, and park service searchers covered another eight miles within the park, scouring the riverbed and moving driftwood and rocks to attempt to uncover any trace of the bodies. Not so much as a scrap of clothing emerged.

On Sunday, September 24, two hundred volunteer searchers covered the length of the river, hoping to bring the final chapter of the Narrows tragedy to a close. Indeed, this became the last day of the search, but no sign of Johnson or Nelson came to light. Sheriff Renouf told the media that he believed the bodies were buried under debris left behind by the storm and flood, and that they were still somewhere at the bottom of the canyon. His statement brought the organized search to an inconclusive but necessary close.

Forty-five years later, in 2006, a man swimming in the Virgin River discovered a bone fragment, the top half of a human skull. He brought it to the Springdale Police, and Chief Kurt Wright thought immediately of the two boys lost in 1961. "That's the only thing that's never really been solved here," he told the Associated Press. "We've had numerous drownings since then in the Narrows, but we've always recovered the victims."

He brought it to the local medical examiner, but they decided not to "reopen old wounds" by contacting the families or testing the fragment, Wright said. At that point DNA testing would have been prohibitively expensive. The bone fragment was stored in a box in the evidence room until another investigator brought it up in 2012, when he learned that the University of North Texas offered free DNA testing to law enforcement—a boon that could clear up at least a portion of a mystery half a century old.

Wright found relatives of the two missing boys in Oregon and Alaska and acquired personal effects that might provide DNA samples. When the results came back from the lab, the skull fragment matched the DNA of Alvin Nelson. The boy's remains were returned to his sister, Doralee Freebairn, for burial in Salt Lake City.

"You'd think after all these years it would be put to rest, but all the stress and frustration just comes right back," said Freebairn. Still, she added, "I find this all very spiritual."

TWO MEN, TOO COLD, TOO FAST

On Wednesday or Thursday, April 21 or 22, 2010, Jesse Scaffidi and Daniel Chidester, two twenty-three-year-old men from Las Vegas, Nevada, began a trip into the Narrows that would test their skills as hikers, wilderness builders, and navigators of rushing water. They told their families that they planned to hike into the top of the Narrows from the Navajo Lake area, ford the Virgin River at its confluence with Deep Creek, and then build a log raft from materials they expected to find in the vicinity. With the raft constructed, they intended to float down the river a distance of fifty miles to Hurricane, Utah, where their journey would come to its triumphant end. They expected to arrive in Hurricane on Saturday, April 24.

It seemed like a great adventure, but none of it was sanctioned by the National Park Service, according to comments park spokesperson Ron Terry made to an Associated Press reporter a few days later. "The Park Service would not have issued a hiking permit in The Narrows because of the danger of high water, nor would officials have approved the plan to build a log raft," the report tells us.

Terry noted that the two men did not attempt to obtain permits or notify any rangers about their plans. Family members told the AP that despite the fact that water in the Narrows is usually very cold in April, the hiker-rafters did not bring cold-water gear or life vests for their journey down the river. "If they had [tried to get permits, they] would not have received a permit due to inappropriate planning and lack of personal safety equipment," a news release from the park informed the media. "At the time, the North Fork of the Virgin River was running about 250 cubic feet per second and the water temperature was around 40 degrees Fahrenheit."

The park's website notes that the Narrows closes when the flow rate is over 150 cubic feet per second (CFS), as well as during spring snowmelt. Swollen with meltwater from a particularly heavy winter snowfall in 2010, the Virgin River was closed to hikers when Scaffidi and Chidester began their trip—and rafting, should anyone have approached rangers with the idea, would have been strictly prohibited.

How fast and powerful is 250 CFS? The answer depends on the waterway itself. Imagine that a cubic foot of water is a box one foot high, one foot wide, and one foot deep, filled with water. Now, choose a spot anywhere on the river, and consider that a fixed point. The number "per second" is a measurement of the number of boxes that move past this fixed point in any given second. So at 250 CFS, 250 of these water-filled boxes move past your selected point in the time it takes to say "One Mississippi." This may be a calm flow in a mile-wide, open river, but in a tight space like the Narrows, where much of the canyon is only twenty to thirty feet wide, that's a lot of boxes of water rushing past a fixed point every second. To maintain that speed, the water must rise within the canyon walls and push through harder and faster than it would at, say, 10 CFS. For two young men riding a makeshift raft on this rushing river through a slim canyon with many twists and turns, 250 CFS would be a deadly speed.

At Zion Adventure Company in Springdale—one of the area's top outfitters and training companies for activities in the Narrows—a sign on the wall provides weather conditions updated daily by staff members. The bottom of the sign includes a "Virgin River Hiking Safety Continuum" chart that clearly indicates the relative danger the river poses at various measures of CFS. At 250 CFS the river is rated as "Very Difficult" for wading—that is, traveling upriver on foot. At 300 CFS the river becomes "Near Impossible" for foot travel. What would the rate be like in the downstream direction?

There is no way to know whether the two adventurers were aware of the dangerous conditions they would encounter, or if they skipped the permitting step because they knew their plan would not receive park approval. Given the risky nature of their intentions, however, it's entirely possible that they had no idea at all.

On Sunday, April 25, when Scaffidi and Chidester did not get in touch with their families to let them know they were safe, a family member contacted the park. The park launched a ground search and used a helicopter to try to locate the men, spending Sunday working their way up the Narrows from the Riverside Walk and down it from the top of the North Fork of the Virgin River.

The first body came to light on Monday morning, April 26, at about 9:00 a.m., near the Gateway to the Zion Narrows. Later that day, at 1:40 p.m., searchers found the body of a second man in the river, more than two miles downstream from the Narrows, near the park shuttle stop at Big Bend. Analysis by the Washington County medical examiner confirmed that these two young men were Scaffidi and Chidester. What exactly killed them—drowning, hypothermia, or a violent encounter with debris in the water—was not determined.

Searchers found no evidence that the men had succeeded in constructing a raft. Without some kind of floating craft, "they would have had to swim much of the Narrows in deep water that is around 40 degrees," Terry told the AP.

READING THE WARNING SIGNS

When two men from Southern California began their hike up the Narrows on Saturday, September 27, 2014, at about 8:00 a.m., the river was flowing at 46 CFS at the Riverside Walk, and rangers had not yet hung signs warning of the potential for flash floods that day.

There were flash flood warnings already in effect, however, for the area surrounding the canyon. Beginning Friday evening, September 26, a storm dropped more than two inches of rain on much of Utah, breaking the day's rainfall records from the Salt Lake City airport all the way to Kodachrome Basin State Park. Roads within Zion National Park flooded with rainwater at various times over the weekend as long, pelting deluges fell and the river crested its banks.

As rain began to fall around 9:30 a.m., the two watched the weather and soon decided to turn back. They were just a quarter-mile from the paved walkway at 10:00 a.m. when floodwaters came barreling down the canyon corridor.

Scrambling for high ground, the two men found perches that kept them out of the water, but they were about two hundred feet apart on opposite sides of the canyon—and the roar of the rushing river made it impossible for them to communicate. They watched and waited for nearly six hours as the water pounded past them at a peak rate of 4,020 CFS, one hundred times harder than when they began their hike a few hours before.

By late afternoon, however, when the river had slowed only to about 1,000 CFS, one of the hikers (whose name was not released) concluded that he needed to move or risk death by hypothermia from sitting still in the chilly canyon. He leapt into the water around 4:00 p.m. and managed to swim out to safety, and he reached a ranger station by 6:30 p.m. to report that his friend, thirty-four-year-old Douglas Yoshi Vo, remained in the Narrows on high ground. He told them that Vo was not injured or in distress, but that he was stranded where he was.

Vo was no stranger to the challenges and unpredictability of the outdoors. His friends called him a Wilderness Explorer (in the spirit of the Disney movie *Up*), one who planned annual camping trips for family and friends. "He thrived on the opportunity to bring his close friends and family, not to his house in Westminster, but to his home in the tents, under the stars," says a tribute to him at YouCaring.com. "How can your sense of adventure not flourish when you have a real-life Wilderness Explorer as your campground leader?"

So Vo's hiking companion felt certain that his friend, who was not injured when last he saw him, would be safe for the short time it would take to bring a rescue party to his location. When the search team arrived at the Riverside Walk, however, they knew immediately that they could not attempt to retrieve Vo until the river's still-extreme pace slowed considerably.

"Rangers arrived at the Narrows, but the river was still flowing at approximately 1,000–1,500 CFS which is too high for them to safely enter the river from downstream," said a news release from the park the following day.

Based on Vo's friend's description of his location, they believed that the remaining hiker was in a relatively safe location, and they planned to hike into the canyon early Sunday morning to be sure he made it to safety.

In the early morning, however, when the other hiker returned to find him, Vo was not in the place his friend had described.

"The rescue effort then turned into a search," the news release noted. Rangers located Vo's body on the riverbank near the Riverside Walk at about 2:00 p.m., roughly a quarter-mile from his last position in the canyon.

"We don't know if he tried to swim as well or if he fell in," said David Eaker, National Park Service spokesperson, to the Associated Press.

Whether Vo fell asleep on his perch and tumbled into the river or attempted an escape and was overcome by the powerful floodwaters, the Narrows turned out to be the last wilderness he would see in his lifetime.

CHAPTER 2

Rising Waters: Incidents in Other Canyons

WHAT IF YOU HAD TO CHOOSE BETWEEN SAVING YOUR BEST friend's life and making sure that five children in your care made it out of the wilderness to safety?

This unimaginable decision was forced upon Mark Brewer, the only adult to survive high waters in Kolob Creek on July 15, 1993. Three adults and five teenage boys began the trek through the canyon at the Lava Point trailhead on July 14, with an adventurous four-day plan to follow Kolob Creek into the Zion Narrows. All of the hikers were members of the Riviera Ward in Salt Lake City, one of the seven wards in the Granite Park Stake of the Church of Jesus Christ of Latter-day Saints. The five boys belonged to a chapter of the Explorer Scouts.

Were it not for Brewer's clarity of decision-making the following day, it was quite possible that none of them would have come out alive.

A narrow canyon sliced through crimson rock by Kolob Creek over thousands of years, the area known as Kolob

Technical Canyons cuts through Zion National Park's northwestern unit and extends northeast of the park into the Deep Creek Wilderness Study Area, a property under the jurisdiction of the US Bureau of Land Management. It's a far less traveled section of the Utah canyon lands than the busy Zion Canyon, making it an area that most visitors miss—even though tourists who don't care for the crowded shuttles in the southern unit can drive Kolob's five-mile scenic road in their own vehicles. It's no less spectacular than Zion's more popular southern unit, with box canyons that rise two thousand feet from the desert floor and glow with the same vermillion and burnt orange tones that make southern Utah so popular with visitors and residents alike.

An information center stands near the entrance to the park's Kolob unit, but beyond it visitors discover a pure, untrammeled wilderness devoid of tourist services. Here the desert remains still except for the distant dashing of waterfalls tumbling over Navajo sandstone ledges. Most hikes in this part of the park lead through natural arches, along the edge of massive formations of crimson rock, interrupted by the shimmer of La Verkin Creek or the press of a startling number of trees, shrubs, and wildflowers. While hiking here can be a rugged experience, the vast majority who walk the twenty miles of trails find Kolob to be a wild, secluded, and peaceful place to wander.

"What is Kolob like?" writes canyoneering expert Tom Jones on his website, CanyoneeringUSA.com.

After a brief walk through the woods, the canyoneer rappels into a pocket garden. A hundred feet further on, the

*canyon starts a drop of 700 feet through numerous pools.
A total of 12 rappels are made, many into crystal clear,
deep green pools followed by short swims and climb-outs
to the next anchor. The canyon is incised deeply, with
delightful grottos and wonderful light reflecting off the
walls. From the bottom of the technical section, the canyoneer can make the long hike out to the Narrows and
the Temple of Sinawava, or can ascend the steep and
strenuous MIA Trail.*

So when Brewer, a thirty-five-year-old advertising executive, and his group—friends Kim Ellis (thirty-seven) and
Dave Fleischer (twenty-eight), and five teens named Shane
Ellis, Chris Stevens, Rich Larson, Mike Perkins, and Josh
Nay—started their second day of hiking with the first ten
rappels down about a thousand feet of cliffs, they expected
some rugged rappelling and a tranquil creek walk at the bottom of a silent canyon. They had obtained the necessary permit from Zion National Park rangers for their expedition,
and among their provisions were inner tubes they would use
to float the last miles through the Narrows to the Temple of
Sinawava. Fleischer had hiked this canyon twice before, so
he had full confidence in what to expect. The three leaders
had even taken the boys camping and canyoneering several
times so they would have the basic skills they needed before
attempting this adventure.

Within minutes, however, the nature of the creek
changed dramatically. "As the canyon narrowed, Kolob
Creek turned into a raging torrent with waters shooting 5
to 8 feet off of waterfalls," the *Deseret News* recounted on

July 22. Despite the hot July weather, the water pounding through the canyon remained icy cold, making it an even greater threat to the eight hikers.

"They had expected some water in the creek canyon; had expected that hiking the streambed would require continued rappelling down a series of waterfalls and past plunge pools," said a report in *High Country News.* "But the water was too fast and too deep."

All three men recognized the danger signs and began to work to provide safe passage for the younger hikers. "I asked Dave if this was what he remembered," said Brewer in an *Outside* magazine story. "He said it wasn't. He said it was ludicrous for us to be in there at all."

To this day, those with canyoneering experience in Kolob Canyon wonder why the party did not turn back at this point.

Fleischer remembered some dry ground ahead, but to reach it, they would have to rappel past four waterfalls—and as soon as they began the attempt to pass the first one, they knew the conditions were even more hazardous than they had supposed. They had to get the boys past a churning whirlpool that swirled at the bottom of the first waterfall.

Fleischer rappelled into the pool to tie ropes for the others to slide over, but "hung on the rope, he had little freedom of movement," the *High Country News* reported. "The boys began yelling that they could see that his backpack strap had slipped around his neck, choking him."

"When Fleischer became entangled in his ropes, Ellis jumped in to assist him," the *Deseret News* said. "The impact of Ellis hitting the water pushed Fleischer out of the whirlpool to safety. But Ellis was now trapped in the whirlpool."

Brewer leapt into the whirlpool to help his friend to safety. "He wasn't in the water more than two minutes," Brewer told the *Deseret News* of Ellis. "But when we got him out, his eyes were dilated and he wasn't breathing."

The two men pulled Ellis from the water, brought him to a logjam, and began cardiopulmonary resuscitation (CPR), working for half an hour to keep him alive. As they worked they realized that Ellis had suffered a blow to the head in his brief time in the raging waters. He lost his life without regaining consciousness.

Fourteen-year-old Shane Ellis, Kim's son, was one of the five boys in the hiking party. With the urgency of their situation now paramount in their minds, Fleischer and Brewer allowed Shane to spend a few minutes with his father before organizing the boys for their next move. They knew the hiking trip was over, but with the force of the rising waters growing stronger, getting the boys back to dry ground had become much more difficult than they had ever planned.

"We were totally committed to not going further, but we had to get to dry ground," said Brewer.

Fleischer knew this part of the canyon well, so he told Brewer and the boys of an alcove ahead where they would be out of the path of the rushing creek. They could wait there, he believed, until they were past the time on Sunday when their families expected them back. He and Brewer secured Ellis's body against a log and guided the now stunned and frightened boys down two more waterfalls. "When they reached the fourth falls, they had been in the water two hours and had made only 50 yards of progress downstream," the *High Country News* said. "They had lost all but two of their backpacks and much of the rope."

The way forward down the fourth waterfall required a fifteen-foot drop and a maneuver around the edge of swirling water in the plunge pool below. Fleischer tied a rope to his backpack and tossed it into the water to judge the strength and direction of the current, and he and Brewer watched as it circled the pool in a constant motion. Then the current grabbed the backpack, and while the rope remained securely fastened to it, they could not pull it out.

Fleischer and Brewer quickly made a plan. Fleischer would jump into the water, retrieve the backpack—which contained most of the food they had brought with them— swim to the side of the pool, and use the backpack as a safety anchor for the rope. Brewer and the boys would then slide down the rope, above the water and out of the current.

At first the plan worked. Fleischer found his way to the backpack, grabbed it, and swam to the side of the pool. As he rested there for a moment, however, his arm slipped and the backpack started to float back into the whirlpool. Fleischer acted on instinct and reached out to grab the pack, and the current sucked him down.

"His strength sapped, Fleischer was himself soon spinning endlessly in the pool," the *Desert News* reported. Brewer watched in horror for his best friend to emerge from the frigid waters, but he never surfaced.

If he jumped into the pool to save his friend, he might also die or become incapacitated—leaving five boys who needed his leadership to come through this ordeal alive. If he stayed on land, Dave Fleischer would die.

In an unimaginable dilemma, Brewer chose to protect and guide the five boys.

"It was very, very difficult," he told the *Deseret News*. "He was such a good friend of mine. But I just knew these boys wouldn't make it without one of us."

Fleischer perished in the whirlpool a few seconds later.

Shattered by watching the deaths of two of their three leaders, the boys suffered from the shock of what they had seen and the terror of staying where they were. They could not turn back and climb the waterfalls. They could not move forward because of the many obstacles the floodwaters had created. Brewer felt no less shocked and horrified, but he knew the boys had no one to turn to now but him. He found his resolve and began to talk.

"I talked to them about being rescued and how we wouldn't be considered lost until Sunday morning," he said. "I laid out the anatomy of a rescue and how it takes time to get organized." This was Thursday; Brewer knew they would be stranded for three long days, and possibly for longer. "My worst fear was that someone else wouldn't make it. I made a pact that everyone else would."

It seemed that everything that made the canyon so appealing to explore now worked against the hiking party as they hunkered down to wait. Their location received barely an hour of direct sunlight each day, and the stone walls and near-freezing water temperature kept the depths of the gorge at a chilly fortyish degrees. Although the boys were all in wet suits, they began to suffer from painful injuries from wearing the suits nonstop for days on end. When night fell—and it came early, with total darkness by 7:30 p.m.—sleep became an elusive blessing. "It was no Motel 6," Brewer told the paper. "We slept in a line of five with those on the ends leaning inward. We had one mummy (sleeping) bag that we pulled over our heads and shoulders. And we laid one boy across our laps."

With so many packs containing most of their food lost in the whirlpool, the boys and Brewer took inventory of their remaining supplies. The menu was meager: "... nine packages of pudding, twelve Kudo candy bars, a couple of fruit roll-ups and nine packages of instant oatmeal. The candy bars provided breakfast for two days; the pudding was supper as each survivor took one bite and passed it on to the next." A box of raisins became a shared meal, with the boys passing the box around in a circle and taking one raisin each until they were gone. "That box lasted twenty minutes," Brewer said.

During the day Brewer came up with projects to keep the boys' minds occupied. They built a rock ledge out of cobbles they found near the creek, making it about eighteen inches wide and six feet long, as a platform on the edge of the water. The boys spent time each day improving their surroundings to increase their sense of security. One day they tore an inner tube into strips that would fit into the top of a mess kit, in hopes of lighting it to make a signal fire for the rescue crews they hoped would arrive on Sunday. In between projects they sang hymns they all knew from church. They watched as the water levels dropped on Saturday, giving them a larger area in which they could dry out their clothing and belongings, and move around to keep warm.

So they remained for four nights until Monday, when the first evidence of a search turned up: the sound of a helicopter overhead. The chopper left and returned twice, but despite their best attempts to attract its attention with leaps, waves, whistles, and calls, Brewer and the boys remained hidden in the darkness. Finally, at about 4:00 p.m., they thought they heard someone whistle back at them. At 4:45 the boys shrieked with relief when an orange rescue rope dropped directly in front of them. "I can't describe the exhilaration and exuberance we felt at that point," Brewer said.

Soon climbers from the National Park Service and the Washington County Sheriff's Office descended and helped the boys up the cliff face, using a winch to lift them to the surface. They camped on top of the mesa that night, well fed and ready to rest under the stars. Early Tuesday morning, a helicopter took them to park headquarters.

Even with the devastating loss of two friends and leaders, Brewer noted days after the experience ended, some good came of the troubled excursion. "Five boys went in there and five men came out," he said. "You could see the personal and spiritual development as time went on. They pulled together and rose to the occasion."

Once the boys were safe, workers went about retrieving the bodies from the canyon. The remains of Kim Ellis came out first on the same day, but the cold water, the high water levels, and the narrow terrain delayed the discovery and removal of Fleischer's body until eleven days later. According to the morning report generated by Zion National Park in July 1994, the effort by searchers working their way up the bottom of Kolob Canyon was "one of the most technically demanding and hazardous retrievals undertaken by the combined county/park SAR team," completed under the direction of district ranger Dave Buccello.

The boys were home again, but their families were left with a single persistent question: Why did the water levels rise so suddenly on July 15, 1993? Weather forecasters had not predicted thunderstorms or heavy rains on that date, so the expedition leaders had not encountered any weather warnings that would deter their trip.

The answer came from the Washington County Water Conservancy District (WCD). A dam at Kolob Reservoir, northeast of the canyon, maintains a constant flow of shallow water through the canyon at any time of the year, so canyoneering visitors find a manageable creek and cooling pools as they move along the bottom. During the growing season, however, the dam serves as part of a sophisticated irrigation system, releasing much heavier flows to the waiting farmlands to the south. The hiking party from Riviera Ward found themselves in the canyon just as the dam released a scheduled irrigation stream.

Outside magazine carried a quote from Ron Thompson, district manager of the Washington County WCD, that said his June records "show that a ranger had been told weeks earlier that the reservoir would be releasing large amounts of runoff into the creek through the spring and summer. 'Anyone familiar with the area should have known that water would be up,' said Thompson."

Who was to blame for this confluence of events became a matter for the courts. In January 1994 the survivors and the families of Ellis and Fleischer filed thirteen claims under the Federal Tort Claims Act, which allows plaintiffs to hold the federal government responsible for specific kinds of wrongdoing. The suit sought a total of $24,556,813 in damages, injuries, and wrongful death. "The claimants say Zion National Park officials failed to warn expedition leaders of unusually large flows of water being released into the canyon from Kolob Reservoir," the *High Country News* reported. "The claims accuse park employees of negligence for issuing a backcountry hiking permit despite the doubly dangerous conditions, and say the agency 'indeed, supported and encouraged the group's expedition into the canyon.'"

The dollar amount represented the total of the lawsuits filed by four of the five boys, Brewer, and Ellis's and Fleischer's families. "The survivors say they suffer flashbacks, reduced ability to concentrate, post-traumatic stress syndrome, and physical discomfort from their prolonged exposure to cold temperatures and water," the *High Country News* reported. "The survivors each want $495,000 for such personal injuries . . . as well as compensation for lost camping equipment and climbing gear—from a $5 water bottle to a $600 sleeping bag."

The surviving spouses each wanted $7.8 million in wrongful death suits, and each of the children sought $925,000.

Not everyone believed the families should bring such suits. "In Utah, where an estimated 70 percent of the population is Mormon, there has been discussion among church members about whether the lawsuit adheres to the teachings of the church," the *High Country News* noted. Outdoor enthusiasts also worried that if public land managers turned out to be culpable for the results of this expedition, wide areas of land could be closed to recreational use in fear that any accident could result in big payouts for the survivors.

After six months of investigation and examination of the case, US Interior Department solicitor Lynn Collins determined that the federal government could not be held liable for the injuries and deaths. "We regret that this unfortunate incident took place and that two members of the hiking party lost their lives," she wrote in a letter to the families' law firm. "However, our review of the information in this matter indicates no evidence of negligence by any employee of the United States."

The survivors and families, continuing to seek restitution, filed another lawsuit against the National Park Service and the water district on August 9, 1994. The suit indicated that they intended to seek a jury trial in the US district court in Salt Lake City. The charge: The ranger who issued the permit did not adequately inform the hikers of the dangerously high water levels, even though the park service and the water district knew the water would be high. This would be a difficult case, however, because the hikers' trip actually began in a part of Kolob Canyon that was outside of the park—and the permit issued to them was for the Narrows, a section of the hike several miles south. "Fleischer's permit, say Park Service officials, was marked with a 'high' danger rating," the *High Country News* reported. "When the danger is measured as 'extreme,' park officials refuse to issue permits. During periods of 'high' danger, rangers can only recommend against expeditions; legally they cannot refuse a permit if other general requirements are met—hikers must have proper equipment and maps and agree not to build fires . . . The Park Service does not assess danger conditions in Kolob Canyon, since it is remote, difficult to access and outside the park."

While Hollywood producers made inquiries about the potential for movie rights to the hikers' stories, a miasma of controversy continued to swirl around this hiking party and the families of the deceased. The Utah canyoneering community squared off in the media, scrutinizing the Explorer Scouts' actions, their equipment, and whether they should have known about the danger before they began the expedition. Reports noted that group members had canceled their hike twice before because of high-water conditions, so they may have felt more determined to make the trip this time despite the warning signs. When they discovered the creek was too high to proceed, some experts suggest that they could have hoisted one leader out of the canyon so he could work from the surface to bring the others out. Some suggest that even if the water was ankle deep to start, the leaders should have known that the flow and level would increase as the canyon narrowed.

Soon the debate about this case became a pitched battle between those who believed the park should take more responsibility for warning people of the dangers of particularly risky activities, and those who called on all risk-takers in parks to accept personal culpability for their own actions. They cited cases throughout the national park system that had led the park service to consider a "no rescue" zone in Denali National Park, and the efficacy of charging climbers fees to offset the $10,000-per-person cost of each rescue from the park's Mt. McKinley, the highest mountain in North America. In Yosemite National Park a man had sued to have a sign placed at the summit of Half Dome, making the obvious point to climbers that they should not stand there during a lightning storm. Outdoor enthusiasts feared that expert climbers and novice hikers alike could be barred from the physical challenges and extraordinary sights that make the parks such popular destinations.

"Most of these tragedies are avoidable," said Charles Cook, then director of the National Center for Wilderness Activities, in the *High Country News* story. "What's upsetting to me is to discover that I can no longer enter a particular area because it has been closed off after a fatality. My freedoms on public lands are infringed by people who were not aware of the risks involved."

In the short term, the most significant change came from Zion management. They asked the Washington County Water Conservancy District to "inform rangers by fax as well as telephone when water is released from the reservoir," according to an *Outside* magazine story. Beyond that the park made no other immediate policy shifts.

Finally, in August 1996, the survivors, the National Park Service, and the Washington County Water Conservancy came to an out-of-court settlement of $2.24 million: $1.49 million from the park service, and $750,000 from the Water Conservancy. The officials involved in the settlement made it clear to media that this "was not an admission of liability," but it did bring the matter to a close.

TRAGEDY IN KEYHOLE CANYON

"We are not a beginning hiking group," Don Teichner, one of the founders of the Valencia Hiking Crew, told potential members on Meetup.com. "A small amount of danger or risk, while still being safe, can also add to a hike's enjoyment."

Teichner and six California-based friends found themselves facing more than a small amount of danger on September 14, 2015, when they descended into Keyhole Canyon in the heart of Zion National Park. The inconspicuous slot canyon, sculpted by eons of flash floods snaking their way between sandstone walls, attracts hundreds of explorers each summer because it's considered a beginner-level canyoneering experience. Five minutes from the Zion–Mt. Carmel Highway and just 1,200 feet long, the canyon requires three short rappels of about thirty feet each to reach the bottom, followed by wading and occasionally swimming through pools created by the Clear Creek tributary that hollowed out this crevice through the sandstone. In some places the canyon becomes so tight that hikers can reach left and right and touch both walls at the same time.

Six of the seven hikers—Gary Favela, fifty-one, of Rancho Cucamonga; Teichner, fifty-five, of Mesquite, Nevada; Muku Reynolds, fifty-nine, of Chino; Steve Arthur, fifty-eight, and Linda Arthur, fifty-seven, both of Camarillo; and Robin Brum, fifty-three, of Camarillo—began their day at an introductory training session led by instructors Laura Dahl and B. J. Cassell of Zion Adventure Company in Springdale. The five-hour class covered canyoneering skills for both Keyhole Canyon and the Subway, a much larger and more challenging slot canyon off of the Narrows. Of the seven in the group, six had never gone canyoneering before (the seventh member, Mark MacKenzie, fifty-six, of Valencia, was the exception)—although they were no strangers to adventure. Six of the members had traveled all over the world to take on challenging hikes together, like Mt. Kilimanjaro in Tanzania and Machu Picchu in Peru. Brum was on her first trip with the group.

"This quick progression from ground school to self-guided canyoneering has played out thousands of times here with relatively few incidents," noted *Outside* writer Grayson Schaffer in a special report for the magazine in May 2016. Commercial guides are not permitted inside the park, so the sixty-thousand-plus people who obtain backcountry permits every year face each canyon's walls on their own. Canyoneers follow an ethic known as ghosting, Schaffer explained, in which they make every effort to leave nothing behind—no ropes, anchors, or other equipment—so each party experiences the canyon in its purest form, "as a mystery to be solved."

MacKenzie went into the park to the visitor center at 7:40 a.m. and bought a permit for the planned Keyhole trip. When he received the permit, the ranger told him that the National Weather Service predicted a 40 percent chance of precipitation, with a possibility of a heavy thunderstorm in the afternoon. The flash flooding risk for the day stood at "moderate," with floods in slot canyons the most likely. "The ranger who handed that permit to that man said, 'I would not go today,'" Zion chief ranger Cindy Purcell told the London *Daily Mail*. "However, the people who go make the choice, they sign the paper that says that it is their safety and their responsibility."

"Less than an hour after the California group received a permit to Keyhole, the weather service raised the chance of rain to 50%," the *Los Angeles Times* reported the following Sunday. "At the Zion visitor center, a ranger wrote on a cardboard sign near the wilderness desk that flash flooding that day was 'probable.' Rangers also informed people verbally when they sought permits."

After the training class, members of the group made contact with family members at home in California. Teichner called his wife, Karen Adams, from the Watchman campground to check on the weather, while MacKenzie texted his son a photo of his surroundings with a bright blue sky in the background. "Maybe Keyhole this afternoon," he said in the text. Later, his phone was found in his truck with a page from the NOAA national weather service still open, listing the Zion forecast for the day as "dry."

At that point there was still only a chance of rain. When the group drove nine miles farther into the park around 2:00 p.m., they lost their cellular phone and data connections, leaving them with no way to see the warning the National Weather Service generated twenty-two minutes later: MOVE TO HIGHER GROUND NOW. ACT QUICKLY TO PROTECT YOUR LIFE. "The warning was publicized through several media sources and posted in all of the park's contact stations," a Zion National Park news release noted. "Canyons were closed to canyoneering."

None of this information reached the seven soon-to-be canyoneers.

The first storm arrived north of the park at about 2:30 p.m. Chances are the Valencia hikers did not see the clouds off to the southwest as they walked in from the parking area to the canyon; perhaps the dark mass was hidden from view by the high sandstone walls of the surrounding landscape. They paused to take a group photo before they entered the slot canyon, a picture of seven relaxed, happy people clad in wet suits and outfitted with climbing and rappelling gear. As they began to move into the slot canyon, a smaller party of three canyoneers arrived at about 4:15, moving at a faster pace than the group of seven. The trio exchanged greetings with the California group and asked to "play through," as the new canyoneers descended the first rappel slowly and with care, cheering one another and "having a great time," according to Jim Clery, who led the smaller group. The three more experienced men slid down the first rappel with ease and moved on. They did not see the seven again.

When the storm arrived at Zion a few minutes later, "It came down hard—rain, hail," Clery told *Outside*. "That's as fast as I've ever seen it change, with as little warning as I've ever seen."

No one can say exactly what happened next to the Valencia group when the storm hit, but weather records show that 0.63 inches of rain fell in the southern part of Zion in less than an hour, beginning at 4:46 p.m. "Rain streaked sideways," the *Los Angeles Times* reported. "Drivers on highways to the north saw dark gray looming over the southern part of Zion."

Clery and his two companions raced through the slot canyon to the culvert under the road, emerging in Clear

Creek and running to their truck. They knew that the party of seven was still in the canyon, and that their chances of survival were slim at best as the rushing current rose above head height. They drove to the nearest ranger kiosk, but rangers already had their hands full with mud-clogged roads, landslides, fallen trees and boulders, and park buses filled with tourists trying to leave the park.

"Rangers noted Keyhole Canyons and several other canyons began to flash flood," the timeline in the park's news release said. "The flow of the North Fork of the Virgin River rose abruptly from 55 cubic feet per second (CFS) to 2,630 CFS in 15 minutes. River levels this high occur approximately once every three years."

Clery's group finally reached the entrance station, where a ranger took down all the information they could provide about the seven hikers trapped in Keyhole.

Once the rain let up, rangers acted quickly to determine whether the party could have somehow survived the flash flood. They found the group's vehicles but saw no evidence that the hikers had emerged from the canyon. "Keyhole Canyon was already flash flooding," the news release continued. "Due to weather at the time and through the evening, it was determined that rescue operations could not be safely initiated." The rangers left a note on the windshield of one of the party's trucks, asking them to check in at a ranger station as soon as they returned.

At 9:00 p.m. rangers went to the canyoneers' vehicles again to see if they had made it back. Nothing appeared to be touched—there was no evidence that they had returned from the canyon.

"In good conditions, the first part of Keyhole can be escaped by scrambling up rock faces or leaving the canyon at an opening near the midway point," the *Los Angeles Times* explained. "But after the route descends deeper—requiring hikers to rappel—there is no turning back until the canyon opens up near Clear Creek and Highway 9." In addition, the three hikers told rangers that the group of seven shared a single rope. This meant that if they had attempted to turn back, they would need to climb out of the canyon one at a time, making any means of escape a slow and deliberate process.

There was no question that this would not be a rescue operation. Park spokesman David Eaker told the *Daily Mail* that "the flooding likely rushed over their heads in moments and carried them miles downstream . . . 'It would be just like a drain, it just funnels down in there very quickly, very fast.'"

On Tuesday morning, September 15, the search and recovery operation began at 7:00 a.m. The water levels remained high in Keyhole Canyon, but searchers followed the canyon's course and peered into it from several loca-tions that were accessible from its rim. They called out for the missing canyoneers but received no response. Walking downstream beyond the mouth of the canyon, they paced along the length of Clear Creek to see if any evidence of the hikers had washed into more open country.

At 1:30 p.m., nearly twenty-four hours after the group entered Keyhole, searchers sorting through debris piles dis-covered the body of Steve Arthur in Clear Creek. Further searching along the creek revealed Muku Reynolds's body at about 4:15 p.m., and Don Teichner's remains in the drainage into Pine Creek at 5:15 p.m.

Meanwhile, between 2:30 and 3:00 p.m., Kaden Anderson, who worked as a canyoneering guide for a local resort, and two friends, newlyweds India and Jay Piacitelli, were about to make the final rappel into Keyhole Canyon on the couple's first-ever canyoneering outing. When they reached the ledge before the third rappel, they discovered a rope hanging down from the ledge to the bottom of the canyon, and they could just see through the dimness that something stuck out of the water below. The shape looked enough like a foot with a shoe on it that it gave all of them pause. "We probably sat there for ten or fifteen minutes," Anderson told Schaffer of *Outside* magazine. "Then I said, 'I'm going to run down and see what's going on.'" He rappelled to the bottom and landed in a muddy pool, and discovered that the shoe he could see was indeed attached to a leg, and the leg to a body. The body turned out to be Gary Favela.

Water levels and weather continued to make the search difficult over the next two days, but more than sixty search and rescue personnel continued in spite of the conditions. On Wednesday, September 16, searchers using cadaver dogs and sifting through piles of driftwood, branches, rocks, and mud found Robin Brum and Mark MacKenzie some distance apart in the Pine Creek drainage. The body of Linda Arthur—the last of the seven—came to light Thursday morning in Pine Creek Canyon; she had traveled the farthest of all on the storm-driven current.

"The most innocuous slot in Zion had produced the worst canyoneering disaster in American history and the

worst accident of any kind in Zion's 97 years," wrote Scha
fer. "The seven people who died in Keyhole Canyon were
experienced hikers. Most of them were not, however, technical canyoneers, well versed in rappelling techniques." This
had never been a life-threatening issue in Keyhole Canyon
before, but as the number of search and rescue missions in
Zion climbs each year—up as much as 29 percent in 2015—
the slot canyons, sheer walls, and summits all become areas
of scrutiny. Schaffer summed it up: "The numbers suggest
that there's something deceptively benign about the desert's
erratic mix of heat, cold, and dryness, interspersed with elec-
trified downpours, that can catch people by surprise."

In the aftermath of the deadliest day in Zion's history,
park officials have begun an examination of the events that
led to the deaths in Keyhole Canyon, and the steps the
park may take to change its own policies regarding access
to canyons, warning systems to reach backcountry hikers,
and assessment of individuals' skills before they take on the
riskiest canyoneering and climbing challenges in the park.
The outcome may include stricter rules around issuing permits, and the requirement that all members of a party hear
weather warnings from rangers or watch a video on the
potential hazards before undertaking risky ventures.

When Easy Trails Turn Deadly

Flash floods can have an effect on safety well beyond the
depths of slot canyons. In a heavy rain, water pours down
over the high cliffs on every side of Zion Canyon, turning
the desert setting into a slippery, sloshy mess and trans-
forming slickrock surfaces into frictionless slides. Waterfalls

:les and expand until they become long, high,
des. Creek tributaries overflow their banks,
ιg streams fill with the debris they gather as
they race ___ g their widened course.

These are the conditions that ten-year-old Michael
Muñoz of Las Vegas, Nevada, and his family encountered on
May 10, 2001, when a spring storm brought heavy rain and
hail to the Canyon Overlook Trail.

On any dry day Canyon Overlook provides a family-
friendly way to see some of the most spectacular views of the
park, beginning just east of the Zion–Mt. Carmel Tunnel
and stretching for half a mile along the edge of Pine Creek
Canyon. Hikers enjoy expansive views of the Switchbacks,
the Beehives, East and West Temple, the Streaked Wall, and
Towers of the Virgin, all icons in the Zion skyline. "There
are lots of hoodoos and wild flowers along the trail that
make it fun for kids, but keep your children close to you and
safe while hiking in Zion," cautions blogger Tanya Milligan,
who writes ZionNational-Park.com, a detailed trip-plan-
ning website. The trail features some steep drop-offs that
add a level of daring and excitement for children, but the
fairly wide path generally provides the required room to pass
these safely.

The Muñoz family walked the half mile to the extraordinary view, and they were on their way back to the parking
area when the rain started. The sudden storm turned the
trail into a perilous mess. As if someone had overturned a
massive pail, rainwater sluiced through a side canyon and
over the trail surface—and to a pair of young boys, wading
through this pop-up stream must have looked like a grand

adventure. They did not realize that the flow could be powerful enough to knock Michael and his younger brother off of the path and over the side of the canyon.

The younger boy managed to grab onto a tree and hold fast until other hikers rescued him. Michael was not so lucky. He tumbled down 250 feet of slope—and then another 150 feet straight down, into the slot canyon formed by Pine Creek.

Park dispatch received the emergency call just after 6:00 p.m., and the search and rescue team responded immediately. A ranger who was also a medic rappelled into the canyon and located Michael, but he discovered exactly what he must have expected: The boy had not survived the long, tumbling fall. The effort to bring the boy's body out of the canyon slowed down when more rain brought another flash flood, but rangers finally completed the dismal job around 11:00 p.m., five hours after the accident occurred.

In a national park with so many fascinating geologic formations and so much dry weather, it can be hard for visitors to comprehend the dangers that can arise when the forecast calls for rain. Zion can change in an instant from a beckoning wilderness to a deadly landscape just by adding water—and hours later, the danger disappears and the trails, canyons, and creek walks become manageable once again. In this park as in so many other undeveloped areas, safety depends not only on skill, training, and preparation, but on timing as well.

CHAPTER 3

Crossing the Neck:
Angels Landing

TOWERING 1,488 FEET ABOVE THE FLOOR OF ZION CAN-yon, Angels Landing provides a 270-degree view of the canyon that no other peak in the park can match. Once known as the Temple of Aeolus, the shape of this spire and the difficult journey required to reach it must have harkened back to a story in the travels of Odysseus, who came upon a floating island known as Aeolia and enjoyed the hospitality of its namesake, the son of Hippotes. When Odysseus and his sailors left the island, Aeolus provided them with a west wind to speed their journey home, and a bag containing winds from three other directions should they require additional assistance. Indeed, those who have stood at the top of this peak have felt the winds from all directions, making the original analogy to Greek mythology quite appropriate.

How the tower's name changed to Angels Landing is the stuff of legend as well. The story goes that in 1916, Frederick Vining Fisher, a Methodist minister from Ogden, Utah, saw the high point from below and exclaimed to his friend and colleague Claud Hirschi, "Only an angel could land on it!" (Fisher and Hirschi named several landmarks in the park, including the Great White Throne.) The name stuck, and visitors from that point forward became fascinated with the option of standing at the top of Angels Landing—a spot reserved only for the winged divine.

In 1926, construction of the trail we still use to reach the summit today became the focus of two park service employees, Thomas Chalmers Vint and Walter Ruesch. Visitors begin the hike using the paved West Rim Trail, and then take the branch that leads gradually upward through a feat of engineering named for Ruesch: Walter's Wiggles. This zigzagging stack of twenty-one switchbacks, each outlined with a low brick barrier, eases the elevation change as hikers make their way through Refrigerator Canyon to the first major viewpoint—the one officially named Scout Lookout.

Colloquially, however, locals know this panoramic overlook by a droll nickname: Chicken-Out Point. Hikers can see not only half of the impressive Zion Canyon from this spot, but also what comes next. Ahead on the trail, a thick chain stretches upward along a slim sandstone fin less than six feet wide. On either side of this ridge, there's a cliff and a sheer drop of more than one thousand feet to the canyon floor below. The chain provides the only handhold, swaying and bouncing as people move up the path to the peak on one side, and down the path to the relative safety at Scout Lookout on the other. (If you'd like to get a sense of what this part of the hike is like, you can take a virtual "eHike" on

, website at www.nps.gov/zion/learn/photosmulti ₁ngels-landing-ehike.htm.)

Ɔne of the problems with the Angels Landing Trail is that it isn't a trail at all, but a series of rock steps so narrow and precipitous that chains to hold onto it have been bolted into the rock face," wrote Julie Sheer in a 2009 blog entry for the *Los Angeles Times*. "This isn't entirely unusual: Think Half Dome [in Yosemite National Park], but instead of a continuous cable-assisted climb, picture narrow rocks barely large enough to stand on in spots—and large gaps between chains. And there are people hiking the trail in sandals, flip-flops and with young children in tow."

Many people take one look at the chain, the meager trail, and the clear air on either side of the ridge and shake their heads, deciding they have come far enough for their own satisfaction. There's no shame in this. One of the most important elements in staying alive in the national parks is to recognize and acknowledge your own limits: Not everyone can hike every trail, nor should you if you know that you are prone to fear of heights, vertigo, or other issues that may cause you to freeze halfway along the ridge or lose your balance. "Angels Landing is one of the most exciting, intimidating, and famous trails in the National Park Service," says Tom Jones in his online Utah Canyoneering Guide. "Many find the final ridge too much, and wait at the 'Widow's Tree' for their companions to return from the summit."

Considering that the trail became accessible to most fearless hikers as far back as 1926, it's remarkable that the first death from a fall off the trail did not occur until 1989—

and what exactly happened to that young man has been shrouded in mystery ever since.

THE BLOODY BACKPACK

On Sunday, April 2, 1989, at about 11:00 a.m., a group of hikers walked into Zion park headquarters and handed the ranger there a backpack spattered with blood. They reported that they had discovered it on Angels Landing, at the peak—so whoever had left it behind had already crossed the ridge and made it to the final viewpoint.

Rangers were immediately dispatched to the trail. When they arrived at the peak, they found a pool of blood at the summit and a trail of blood spots on the north edge, but they could not see a body from there. It took a helicopter to finally locate the owner of the backpack around 4:15 p.m.—a body lying on a ledge about 150 feet down the side of the sandstone pillar. A recovery crew removed the body the following day and discovered that the man had a large hole in his forehead, one that "could be a gunshot wound or could have resulted from injuries sustained in a fall," according to Washington County medical investigator Al Boyack.

"We've got a real mystery on our hands," he told the *Spokane Chronicle* on Tuesday, April 4.

Authorities were able to determine the man's identity as the investigation continued. His driver's license gave his name as Jeffrey Robert Dwyer, a twenty-eight-year-old resident of Sandpoint, Idaho, and they found that Dwyer was traveling with two other people on a seven-week trip through the western United States and Mexico. Dwyer had gone out on his own, without his friends, early Saturday afternoon, and they had not seen him since. Another hiker saw Dwyer alone later on Saturday.

"There's a lot of injury to the head," Chief Ranger Bob Andrew told the media, "but what we're concerned about is all the blood on the top of Angels Landing. We're awaiting the autopsy to determine the cause of death. Right now we're just calling it a fatality."

The results of the autopsy did nothing to solve the mystery, however. The examination showed that Dwyer died from "massive head injuries," Washington County sheriff Glenwood Humphries told the media. He emphasized that investigators were "still awaiting the results of additional medical tests before ruling whether Dwyer's death was accidental, a homicide or a suicide."

Andrew said that cause of death remained under investigation, adding, "There's enough suspicion because of the amount of blood we found that we've ruled it a suspicious death." Sheriff's deputies also noted that they had found a half ounce of marijuana in Dwyer's pocket, though no reports drew any conclusion from this.

Remarkably, this was the last attention the media paid to this questionable death in the park. None of the local papers or the national wire services followed up to discover what conclusions these investigations may have confirmed.

All suspicious deaths in national parks come under the auspices of the Federal Bureau of Investigation. I made a request under the Freedom of Information Act to see the file on the Dwyer death, and I was surprised at the response: There is no file on Jeffrey Robert Dwyer. The Washington

County Sheriff's Office responded to my request for information on the investigation as well, but the office's files only go back to 1997. There's no record of a continued investigation or the results.

So what happened to Dwyer? Did he reach the summit, fall and hit his head, and roll off the cliff? Did someone strike him and run—and if so, to what end? Or did he purposely take his own life? No one knows. The case has long since gone cold, and the incident remains a mystery.

ZION'S FIRST RAPPELLING ACCIDENT

Nearly eight years passed before another event on Angels Landing resulted in a death.

On January 1, 1997, thirty-six-year-old John Michael Christensen decided to celebrate the new year with a solo climb of Angels Landing. A skilled climber, Christensen had all of the appropriate technical gear with him, and he chose to take the route known as the Prodigal Sun, one of the rock faces of the tall sandstone peak.

While the *Deseret News* called this a "relatively easy route," Prodigal Sun takes an unrelentingly vertical approach to the peak. It involves scaling sheer rock faces, scrambling through loose rock and dirt, finding footing over the lips of arches and diagonal pitches, and belays from one anchor to the next along ledges less than a human foot wide. Some of the area's lead climbers have set pitons to help others work their way up the rock face, but most consider this a two-day climb today, with the first day spent setting up the first three pitches and coming back down to camp. With this preparation completed, climbers can spend the second day "blasting" all the way up the wall to the top. The climb can take from dawn to dusk on a summer day, so with the shortened daylight on the first of the year, Christensen spent at least part of it climbing in the dark.

That's why no one saw Christensen climbing the peak, but investigators believe that he made it to the top without mishap. Once he stood at the Angels Landing viewpoint, he had two choices: He could take the long walk down the snow-covered path—the one used by day hikers to reach the landing the more conventional way—or he could go back down the way he came. The rappel back to the parking area probably looked more appealing to a man who had just conquered the rock face.

The accident took place on the way down.

When Christensen did not contact his family at the appointed time, his family reported to the park that he was missing. It took searchers only a short time to find his body at the base of the peak.

"There's no 100 percent certainty because there were no witnesses and it was in darkness," National Park Service investigator David Buccello told reporters, but the ropes and rappel device Christensen was using when he fell indicated that he was on the descent. "The gear harnessed to the victim suggested he rappelled off the end of one of the two ropes he was using."

The Associated Press reported that Christensen "employed two 200-foot ropes, one 11 millimeters thick, the other 8 millimeters. Both were used for the rappel in which their ends were tied together and fed through anchors secured to the rock," giving Christensen a total of four hundred feet of rope length for the rappel. This arrangement requires extra care during the rappel, however, because "the smaller rope will feed through the rappel device faster than the fatter one, because its smaller surface area produces less friction." Some thirty feet of rope was still attached to the rappel device when Christensen was found.

Buccello suggested a second possibility: Christensen may have been struck by a falling rock, which in turn made him let go and fall. Either way, the investigator speculated that Christensen had fallen more than six hundred feet.

"John loved the outdoors," Christensen's obituary in the *Deseret News* read, "and he loved being with his family." Before his death he had been serving as the young men's president in the Edgemont Sixteenth Ward of the Church of Jesus Christ of Latter-day Saints. He and his wife were raising five children.

No Unnecessary Risk

Some deaths on Angels Landing occur out of sheer bad luck—not because people underestimated their fear of heights or attempted to scale a precipitous wall. Georg Sender, age sixty-three, came to Zion from Illertissen, Germany, with Rotel Tours of Germany—one of thousands of tourists from countries around the world who visit Utah's national parks every season. It's no surprise that he would choose to hike up the trail to Angels Landing to see one of the most magnificent views in the American West, nor is it particularly unusual for someone to stray off the trail a few feet to get a closer look at an interesting butterfly or to catch an early glimpse of the panorama.

In Sender's case, however, the momentary lapse proved disastrous. He tumbled down a slope and fell roughly fifteen feet. Exactly what injuries he suffered were not detailed in the park's morning report the following day, but the account of the incident, written by Zion staff member Tom Haraden, gave a gripping description of the August 2, 2000, accident scene: "Several EMT's and a Swiss emergency room physician were nearby and provided immediate medical assistance, including CPR. The latter was terminated after 45 minutes after consultation with the physician on scene and medical control at Dixie Regional Medical Center. A hiker in the vicinity used his cell phone to call for help, and park personnel were dispatched to the scene; an NPS trail crew working nearby was first to arrive. The body was removed by helicopter. Counselors were on scene to provide assistance to witnesses and family and conduct a CISD briefing for responders." Most accident victims do not have the benefit of the immediate medical attention Sender received; it was his misfortune that his injuries were too severe to respond to this intervention.

The death of Mark Ertischek, a sixty-year-old attorney for the municipality of Anchorage, Alaska, might not have received national media coverage in an average week, but the week including his death on June 9, 2007, was far from average. Zion experienced its first-ever series of three deaths in the space of a few days, of which Ertischek—who collapsed with a heart attack while walking the trail on the approach to Angels Landing—was the third. (Another of the three, Barry Goldstein, is detailed later in this chapter; Keith Biedermann's fall in Heaps Canyon is in chapter 5.)

"Park officials say a vacationing firefighter was the first on the scene and began to administer CPR," the Associated Press story tells us.

Tiffany DeMasters of *the Spectrum*, the newspaper of St. George, Utah, spoke with public information officer Tom Haraden to find out more. Haraden said that while Ertischek was hiking alone, several people on the trail saw him fall to the ground. "When he collapsed, there was no heartbeat and no pulse," Haraden said. "We did CPR for about 50 minutes until DRMC told us to cease."

Ertischek had provided his legal expertise to the State of Alaska Attorney General's Office and the state's Human Rights Commission, making his death a fairly high-profile one in Alaska and beyond.

FALL FROM SCOUT LOOKOUT

Dorothy Kaiser, a sixty-six-year-old visitor from Joshua Tree, California, left her hotel room at Zion Lodge on Sunday, January 19, 2003, and drove to the nearby Grotto parking area. She left her vehicle and started up the trail to Angels Landing—a trail that likely had some icy patches along its 2.4-mile length, but that may not have daunted someone hardy enough to visit Zion in winter on her own. After a fairly energetic hike with an elevation gain of about 1,100 feet, she reached Scout Lookout—a good place to stop and admire the view well above the floor of Zion Canyon.

What exactly happened next has never been determined, but Kaiser did not return to her room at Zion Lodge.

On Monday, January 20, when Kaiser did not check out on time, Zion Lodge staff went to her room late in the day and discovered that her belongings were still inside. The lodge contacted park headquarters, and dispatchers alerted the night patrol rangers to begin looking for her vehicle. The rangers discovered it parked at the Grotto. When it was still there the following morning, a search team set out on the West Rim Trail to trace Kaiser's most likely route after she left her car on Sunday. They reached Scout Lookout, peered over the edge, and spotted "some type of personal gear at the base of Scout Lookout," according to the park's morning report.

The team radioed this news to dispatch, and a second search team made its way to the base of the peak. There they found the body of Kaiser, who had fallen nine hundred feet from Scout Lookout.

The matter went to the Washington County Sheriff's Office for further investigation, but that office tells me that there is no record of any findings.

Only Kaiser knew exactly what happened on that chilly January afternoon. Perhaps she stepped on a patch of ice and slid over the edge. Perhaps—and this seems more likely—she intended to end her life . . . and if so, perhaps her motives are none of our business.

THE BET

The newspaper accounts were surprisingly terse about the death of young Kristoffer Jones, a fourteen-year-old boy from Long Beach, California, on June 25, 2004. The Associated Press reported that Jones and his Boy Scout troop were "at Angels Landing, a popular but steep hiking spot in the southern Utah park, when he fell off a cliff Friday afternoon . . . A search and rescue crew had to rappel down the cliff to get to the body, which was recovered Saturday morning."

Park spokesperson Ron Terry said that the incident was under investigation, "but we don't know the cause at this time."

They soon found a more harrowing chain of events than anyone would wish to discover.

The Washington County Sheriff's Office and the National Park Service revealed that Jones went out onto a slim ledge eight hundred feet above Zion Canyon and well off the Angels Landing trail to scratch his name into the side of the cliff.

He did this to impress a group of boys he had just met on his visit to Provo, while he stayed with his grandmother and his uncle, Rene Doria, as he often did during the summer. Doria had approved his nephew's participation in a trip to Zion organized by the Bonneville Third Ward of the Church of Jesus Christ of Latter-day Saints, along with about forty Scouts, with the assumption that the group would have adequate adult supervision by ward and Scout leaders to keep them all safe.

Once in the park, the group split into four groups of ten. Somehow, a group of four or five boys including Kristoffer broke away from the larger group as they approached the peak of Angels Landing, and they became separated from their leader. The other boys dared Kristoffer to go out on a ledge some 1,200 feet above the canyon floor and write his name on the cliff face. They sweetened the deal with a wager of five dollars against his ability to do it.

Kristoffer took the bet. "Boy Scouts are taught to eschew risky behavior, but none of the Scouts who knew of the bet tried to stop Kristoffer from collecting," a story in the *Salt Lake Tribune* noted. "According to investigative reports, one Scout who watched Jones crawl onto the ledge simply told the boy, 'Don't die.'"

The other participating boys are not named in the report, but Chief Deputy Rob Tersigni told *Tribune* reporter Matthew D. LaPlante that photographs taken by a witness show "several boys standing on a ledge behind Kristoffer on Angels Landing." The witness told police he saw the boys running around and jumping between rocks—all without an adult Scout leader present. Later, the same witness "saw three of the Scouts walking back down the trail and overheard one of them say, 'He's probably hurt or dead.'"

The boys had left the trail and were hundreds of feet beyond where it was considered safe to go. "According to the report, Kristoffer was about six feet from the nearest Scout and was scooting along a steep slope when he lost his footing," the *Tribune* said.

Only one of the boys said that he actually saw Kristoffer fall. Several, however, heard him scream. Even then, the boys did not run for help immediately—instead, they linked arms and formed a chain to see if they could see where Kristoffer had landed. By the time an adult arrived at the top of Angels Landing, the damage was long since done.

Several weeks later, when the sheriff's report of the investigation landed on the desks of the Boy Scouts' Orem-based National Parks Council, executives knew they had a problem that required action. Unit-level Boy Scout executive

Gaylun Smith told the *Tribune* that he would "find out who did what . . . It's really sad for the boys who did this, because even if no action is ever taken, they will have to live with this—and they have a lot of life left to live." He noted that one of the leaders who had been on the Zion trip with the Scouts had "changed callings" of his own volition because of what happened to Kristoffer.

The sheriff's report also made Kristoffer's family begin to consider legal action against the Scout troop. Two years later, on June 14, 2006, Ruth Jones, Kristoffer's mother, filed a lawsuit against the Boy Scouts of America, the Utah National Parks Council, and the Church of Jesus Christ of Latter-day Saints claiming negligence on their part in her son's death.

Lynn Harris, the Provo attorney representing Jones, had served as a Scoutmaster himself. "My first allegation in the suit was, who was the idiot who decided to take 40 Scouts to the top of Angels Landing?" he told the *Los Angeles Times*. "They are kids. They do stupid things."

While the *Times* reported that a settlement was reached in the case, the court ordered that the terms be sealed.

FALLING FROM THE NECK

Perhaps the increasing popularity of Zion National Park drew more hikers to Angels Landing in the latter half of the twenty-first century's first decade, or perhaps the availability of information about the strenuous hike heightened its appeal. With more hikers came more opportunities for people to misjudge the very real danger involved in crossing the slim ridge to reach the viewpoint just beyond it.

Bernadette Vander Meer was an experienced hiker, as a cousin who posted to the National Parks Traveler blog on August 30, 2006, made clear. "My cousin Bernadette had been hiking from a very young age," she wrote. "She new [sic] about the dangers."

Vander Meer worked at the New York New York Hotel and Casino in Las Vegas, led worship and sang at the New Song Christian Church there, and lived "a life painted in love," as her family expressed on August 23 in the *Las Vegas Review-Journal*. "She loved family, friends, nature, music, and performing on stage," the notice continued.

At dawn on Tuesday, August 22, 2006, twenty-nine-year-old Bernadette and her husband, David, rode bicycles into Zion to the Grotto parking area and began their hike on the West Rim Trail to Angels Landing. They passed Scout Lookout, and began their crossing of the neck when something went wrong. Whether Bernadette had a spell of vertigo, lost her grasp of the chain meant to provide a sturdy handhold, or bobbled her footing, or a rock gave way underfoot, we will never know for certain. What we do know is that she fell to the canyon below.

David called 911 from his cellular phone, and the emergency dispatch notified the park at 6:30 a.m. Search and rescue teams responded quickly. Bringing a helicopter in from Page, Arizona, they spotted Bernadette on a talus slope about 1,200 feet below Angels Landing and notified the ground rescue team of her location. It was 4:00 p.m. before they brought her body out of the canyon.

Washington County sheriff's chief deputy Rob Tersigni told the *Deseret News* that the sheriff's office was treating the death as an accident. "The investigation is not complete yet," he said on the day of Vander Meer's death. "We're leaning towards an accidental fall, but we're still following up on it." Evidence pointed investigators to the eventual conclusion that this was indeed nothing more than a tragic accident.

A year later, another fall claimed the life of a fifty-three-year-old man hiking with a large group of family and friends. This time, witnesses actually saw the victim on his way across the neck, standing close to the edge—and then disappearing over it.

Dr. Barry S. Goldstein and his family were visiting from Creve Coeur, a suburb of St. Louis, Missouri, to celebrate a wedding that was to take place the following day.

"We were sitting there and couldn't believe what we were watching," said Mike Farley, who was eating lunch with a group of teenage boys and other adults at a nearby peak on June 8, 2007, when a man within their range of sight suddenly vanished over the edge. "It was a sheer dropoff. There were no second chances when he went off."

Farley immediately dialed 911. "They had left ten minutes before us and were crossing the narrow neck," he told the *Deseret News* later that day. "The guy had been standing near the edge . . . the man who was next to him before he fell later told me that he [Goldstein] was goofing off near the edge and the ground crumbled as he stepped back. We could see him fall—just like that he was gone."

Zion Dispatch also received a call from Goldstein's family members at 11:55 a.m., and rangers immediately responded. They searched at the base of the cliff and found the body quickly, confirming that the fall had been fatal. "It is estimated that Goldstein fell approximately 1,000 feet to his death," the park's news release said.

While friends and coworkers in St. Louis were shocked to hear of Goldstein's death, "no one was surprised to hear it happened while he was hiking along the edge of a towering cliff in a national park," the *St. Louis Post-Dispatch* noted on June 11, 2007.

Friends knew that the well-liked anesthesiologist loved to be outside, and that he exercised daily and kept in shape. Goldstein visited Vail, Colorado, twice a year to hike the mountain trails, according to Dr. Christopher Felling, one of his partners in private practice at Ballas Anesthesia. "Hiking was his thing," Felling told the *Post-Dispatch*.

Goldstein and his family had just moved to a larger house in Town and Country, Missouri, one they had spent time gutting and rehabilitating. He had joined the private practice just five years earlier after working as the head anesthesiologist at the Des Peres Square Surgery Center. "Co-workers described Dr. Goldstein as an excellent doctor," the paper said. "He was funny, easygoing, and enjoyed wine."

Like Bernadette Vander Meer, Goldstein had plenty of hiking experience, and he knew what to expect at the top of Angels Landing. The fact that knowledgeable, athletic hikers have plunged to their death from this peak says a great deal about the need for caution and self-awareness when daring yourself to cross the neck.

Nancy Maltez of Glendora, California, also was no stranger to a challenging trail. "She was an experienced hiker," her sister posted to the National Parks Traveler website on August 10, 2009. Maltez had reached the summit of Angels Landing with her husband and three children—ages fourteen to twenty—on Sunday morning, August 9, 2009, just as she and her family had done a number of times before. This time, however, she took a wrong step while crossing a portion of the trail known as the "saddle area" on the way to the summit, and lost her footing.

"I am told [this trail] was one of their favorites," her sister continued. "By all accounts she simply stumbled and fell. She was a very grounded person so I am sure there would have been no horseplay up there."

Search and rescue crews located Maltez's body before noon, and the park and sheriff's office closed the trail for a few hours as they completed their investigation. Meanwhile, discussion on hiking, canyoneering, and park enthusiast websites began to buzz about Angels Landing and the mounting number of fatalities there in recent years. Some called for the trail to be closed permanently. Others recommended that warning signs be posted, including a sign that would list all the recent deaths. Many commented that untold thousands of people hiked the trail each year without incident, and that the trail was "safer than a car ride."

Julie Sheer of the *Los Angeles Times* noted, "As for Angels Landing restrictions, of course the trail should not be closed, or have a snack shop at the top . . . I do think some additional signage wouldn't hurt. It might send a signal to casual hikers and make them stop and think before proceeding."

Not quite four months later, on November 27, another hiker fell from the peak.

Tammy Grunig and her husband, Michael, had pur-
chased a home in St. George with the goal of moving there
from their residence in Pocatello, Idaho, one day to retire.
They split their time between the two homes as Tammy
worked in audiology and speech pathology at Portneuf
Medical Center in Pocatello, and Michael held a job with
ON Semiconductor there. Tammy also served as an affili-
ated clinical staff member at Idaho State University, and she
worked with a home health organization as well.

They had just returned from spending Thanksgiving
in Las Vegas with Michael's mother and younger brother,
when Tammy decided to go hiking in Zion. Rick Grunig,
Michael's brother, told the *Idaho State Journal* that Tammy,
who was fifty years old, had recently focused on getting into
shape and losing some weight. "She talked about [hiking] to
my mom during Thanksgiving," Rick said. "She's not a real
big hiker, but she had been on Angels Landing before. She
was basically trying to get herself fit again. She had dropped
about 60 pounds, if not more. She was looking really good."

Tammy set off to hike alone while Michael ran some
errands. They made plans to meet up at the park later that
afternoon.

When Michael arrived at the park, Tammy was not back
from her hike. As the afternoon wore on, he became more
and more worried and finally went to the ranger station to
report that she was late. "Then about an hour and a half after
he got there, he heard from [park rangers] that a woman had
fallen to her death," Rick said.

"The fall of approximately 1,000 feet occurred on the
north side of the popular Angels Landing while Mrs.

Grunig was hiking the popular route," the park's news release announced on November 30. "The fall was first reported by a 911 call from another hiker's cell phone; St. George Police Dispatch Office received the call at approximately 2:10 p.m." The park sent out a search and rescue team, who recovered Grunig's body by 6:30 p.m.

Five months later to the day, one more woman plunged to her death—but this time, the thousand-foot fall took place at Scout Lookout, before the hike across the neck. Park dispatch received a call at 4:20 p.m. on April 27, 2010, that the woman had fallen. She "was seen sitting on the edge of Scout Lookout," the *Salt Lake Tribune* reported. "When she stood up . . . [she] lost her balance. She plummeted about 1,000 feet."

Search and rescue personnel located her body later that evening. When they recovered it the following morning, they found that she had no identification with her, so no positive identification could be made right away—and no one contacted the park looking for her.

"Park rangers are looking for vehicles that have been left unattended and are investigating whether any guests staying in the park or in nearby Springdale had not checked out when they expected to in an effort to confirm the woman's identity," the *Salt Lake Tribune* reported on April 29.

Their search eventually bore fruit. A local hotel reported that a female guest had not checked out on time, and that her belongings were still in her room. Police found her driver's license in the room and matched the photo of the guest with the victim: she was Regine Milobedzki, age sixty-three, of Upland, California. Even with this information in hand, however, it still took law enforcement several days to locate and reach family members to notify them of the accident.

It had been a rough week for staff and search teams at Zion. Just a few days before, two men—Daniel Chidester and Jesse Scaffidi, both twenty-three—planning to build a raft and float the Virgin River through the Narrows had died before they could attempt their feat. (You'll find their story in chapter 1.)

ANGELS LANDING TODAY

With a deadly fall every few months from 2007 to 2010, and a number of additional rescues that did not end in fatalities—including saving those who started across the slim fin and froze midcrossing—park officials knew that it was time to make Angels Landing safer for hikers.

In the spring of 2011, the last half mile of the hike got a limited but effective safety makeover. "The park service installed more chains, which hikers can grip like a stairway railing as they walk," the *Salt Lake Tribune* reported. "The park service also carved more steps in the rock."

Now a sign near the trailhead gives some hikers pause before they begin the crossing. It warns them that six people have died from falls on the trail since 2004. "The route is not recommended during high winds, storms, or if snow or ice is present," the sign continues.

The changes appear to be working. As of this writing, no one has died on Angels Landing since 2010.

CHAPTER 4

The Edge of Forever:
Falls from High Places

EUGENE CAFFERATA, A NINETEEN-YEAR-OLD FROM ST. Louis, Missouri, had some exciting plans for the summer of 1930: He and his friend, John Faust, would accompany John's mother, Rose, on a tour of the American West. Rose and Eugene's mother, Christine Cafferata, had been classmates at St. Louis University years earlier, and when Christine's husband died in 1922 and the family gave up the restaurant of which he was the proprietor, it became harder for them to take elaborate vacations.

On Tuesday, July 8, Rose, John, and Eugene took a horseback ride through Zion Canyon and explored some of the trails. Eugene realized that he would be stiff and sore the next day from spending time on horseback if he didn't take a walk before turning in that night. He bade his friends a good afternoon, said he would be back for dinner, and started up the trail to Emerald Pools, just a short distance from Zion Lodge.

That was the last anyone saw of Eugene until two days later.

In the first half of the twentieth century, the relatively easy Emerald Pools trail offered a compelling side trip, a steady but navigable climb up to the summit of neighboring Lady Mountain. "Today's obscure route to the summit of this Zion landmark was once a popular and maintained trail, equipped with chains and other safety devices," Tanya Milligan writes on her extensive website, ZionNational-Park.com. "Completed in 1924, this amazing route up the steep mountainside was the first trail constructed by the park leading to one of the rims." The route featured more than 2,000 feet of cable and 1,400 carved steps, making it an adventurous climb for tourists looking for a challenging hike. (Today all the cables are gone and the route is no longer maintained, so this has become a technical route for experienced climbers.)

Once he started up the Middle Emerald Pool trail, Eugene reached the trail to Lady Mountain and decided it was just strenuous enough for his post-ride stretch. He worked his way up the trail to the summit, climbing about 2,650 feet in just 1.9 miles until he reached the top at 6,945 feet. Here, no doubt, he enjoyed the view for a time before he signed the trail registry at about 7:30 p.m. and started back down the trail as the sun sank lower in the western sky.

When Eugene did not return for dinner and still had not arrived well after dark, Rose and John alerted rangers that he was missing. "Rangers concentrated their search on the canyons and thick brush of the vicinity," the *St. Louis Post-Dispatch* reported, "thinking he must have altered his plans after leaving the lodge." When this produced no evidence of Eugene's whereabouts, they widened their search. His signature in the trail registry, discovered two days later, became the first clue to what had happened to the young man.

Now the searchers retraced their steps down the steep trail, and soon the fifteen-member team led by Chief Ranger Joseph Holley spotted something in a crevice not far from the top of the mountain. It became clear that Eugene had wandered off of the trail in the dark and fallen over the ledge, tumbling about fifty-five feet until he fell into the crack.

The examination of his body determined that Eugene broke a rib in his fall, and the bone penetrated one of his lungs. "He probably lived for some time after the accident," an account in the *Ogden Standard-Examiner* said.

THE FATAL LAST STEP

No matter how much spectacle each viewpoint in Zion National Park delivers, someone in the park's history has wished to see just a tiny bit more. The desire to get just a little closer to the edge of a cliff has proved fatal for at least sixteen people, including Eugene Cafferata, making a slightly more expansive look downward or outward—or a carelessly placed footfall—the last act in their lives.

All of the fifty-nine national parks have established trails, many of which feature barriers, guardrails, fences, or railings to keep people on the right side of safety. In Zion many of the most frequented trails have no such divisions between hikers or climbers and clear air. It's up to the visitor, then, to acknowledge that the park has placed its maintained trails along potentially hazardous routes, and that staying on these routes, while not a perfect guarantee of safety, certainly improves the odds of surviving the experience.

Zion features a number of trails that follow the top edge of high sandstone walls or narrow ledges carved by millions of years of weather and erosion. Hiking these can be an exhilarating experience, both because of the stunning formations and landscapes that surround the trail, and because of the potential for danger just a few feet or even inches away. This is a park that informs the visitor: We know you're a responsible adult, and that you respect the limited boundaries we've set for you. Now, take it from here. Keep an eye on your children so they don't wander too close to the edge. Watch your own steps and be sure you're in the safest zone.

Not all visitors understand their personal role in protecting their own lives, however, and some who cross the line do not survive. Such was the case with Lane Kelton Cottrell, a seventeen-year-old employee of the park company who worked in the kitchen at Zion Lodge. Cottrell went hiking in the vicinity of the Great White Throne trail with two companions on September 4, 1951. They headed up Mountain of the Sun and reached the summit, and were on their way back down when Cottrell decided that he wanted to take his time down the route instead of keeping up with his friends. The other two went on ahead, assuming that Cottrell would meet them at the lodge later that evening.

When Cottrell was not back by dark, the two other hikers contacted rangers. Their ten-hour search through the night finally revealed that Cottrell had fallen off a ledge when he strayed from the trail. He fell forty feet into a small canyon between Mountain of the Sun and the neighboring

Deer Trap Mountain, where he remained wedged 1,500 feet above the canyon floor until the search team found him at about 6:00 a.m. on September 5. Eerily, Cottrell's watch had stopped at 8:10 p.m., roughly the time that he had most likely perished from the fall.

INTRODUCTION TO SLICKROCK

If you've never hiked in Utah, the concept of slickrock may conjure up images of wet boulders in a streambed or vertical rock faces worn smooth by centuries of weather events. In sandstone country, slickrock isn't actually slick at all in dry conditions—in fact, its surface creates enough friction to feel like coarse, sixty-grit sandpaper against palms and knees. A slickrock trail can offer fairly stable hiking and technical work in the driest seasons, making otherwise challenging trails seem a little easier than expected.

When the summer rains arrive, however, moss can take hold on horizontal sandstone surfaces, turning otherwise rough rock into a surface as slippery as ice. This is what caused Kelly Hilton, a seventeen-year-old boy from Murray, Utah, to slide off the trail and 125 feet down into the canyon on August 5, 1959.

Hilton was the third cook at the Zion Park Inn (now Zion Lodge) that summer, and he would have been a senior at Granite High School in Murray that fall. The group with whom he was hiking—including coworkers Robert Browning, seventeen, and Jimmy Iverson, fifteen, and Zion Park Inn manager Theron Toogood—chose Natural Bridge Canyon as their target destination. Instead of taking the well-established route that began near the entrance to the

Zion-Mt. Carmel Tunnel, however, the boys chose an abandoned trail near the park's south entrance, one that had not been maintained since the 1930s. Back then, park management had fastened rope ladders to the rock so that climbers could pull themselves up the vertical rock faces and over steep ledges. The ladders had long since been removed.

The four hikers left Zion Park Inn at 4:00 a.m. to begin their hike. At about 7:10 a.m. Browning and Iverson heard something up ahead—a cry for help, and a rush of falling gravel. "I heard him slip and thought it was a rock falling," Browning told United Press International. "Then I saw Kelly flying through the air. I heard him moan once as he hit the first time. Then we lost sight of him."

They rounded the next bend and saw "a pair of loose-fitting loafers and a place where the moss had been scraped from a rock," as Frank Jensen of the *Salt Lake Tribune* reported on August 6. Kelly Hilton was nowhere in sight, and the thick brush below the ledge made it impossible to see where he had gone.

Toogood ran for help as the boys began searching for their friend. He returned with a search team including Chief Ranger Fred Brueck, who lowered himself into the gorge on a rope and found Hilton in minutes. "The youth was lying with his head twisted under his chest," Jensen reported. "The body had fallen over a vertical 75-foot cliff and rolled another 50 feet. He apparently had landed on his head, dying instantly."

Rangers recovered the body and brought it out of the gorge at 1:50 p.m.

When Children Fall

Eleven-year-old Dana Harrison of Logan, Utah, probably felt fairly confident on his way up the Lady Mountain trail on June 21, 1962, enough so that he left his father, Thede Harrison, and his two older brothers, Max and Richard, to head back to the family camp on his own. What exactly happened next will never be known, but when his brothers and father returned to camp after their hike, at about 12:30 p.m., and discovered that Dana had not arrived, they went back up the trail to try to find him. It was only when their efforts failed that they alerted park rangers to the fifth grader's disappearance. By then it was 4:00 p.m.

Dana had fallen about fifty feet down a rock cliff at about noon and had survived, although he was unconscious—so no cries for help alerted the thirty-member search and rescue crews to his location. Even so, the teams located Dana at about 7:00 p.m., less than three hours after their efforts began. The boy had already lain unconscious on the mountain for about seven hours, and it took another five hours for the skilled crew to reach him at the base of Lady Mountain, secure him to a stretcher, and carry him out of the remote area over steep, rocky terrain. They discovered that he had significant head injuries, including a crushed skull, but he was breathing—a sign of hope.

Once he realized the boy was alive, Chief Ranger James Felton contacted Dr. Garth Last in Hurricane, about fifty miles south of the park, to meet the rescue team at Lady Mountain with an ambulance. It was well past midnight when Dr. Last had his first opportunity to examine Dana and administer first aid. "The boy survived nearly fourteen hours from the time of the fall until he was discovered and carried by litter down the steep mountain," the *Star Valley Independent* told readers. "But he died as the rescue party reached the base of the mountain and the ambulance. Oxygen and respiration equipment failed to revive him."

Almost six years passed before another young child met his fate in a fall, but this one took place on a trail not too far distant. On March 3, 1968, Robert Casalou and his friend Gerald Gifford, both of whom were thirteen and both visiting from North Las Vegas, set out on the Emerald Pools trail to make it all the way to the top. When they reached Upper Emerald Pool, they could enjoy the sight of an eighty-foot waterfall swelled with late winter snowmelt, and at least partially encased in huge columns and formations of solid ice.

At about 2:00 p.m., they came to a ledge near the falls and sat down to take in the view. Casalou inched closer for an even better look, forgetting in that moment that the sandy surface would act as a glide against rocks wet with spray from the roaring falls. Momentum took him, and he plunged over the side of the ledge.

Gifford, stricken with panic, ran the entire one and one-quarter miles to the trailhead near Zion Lodge. He flagged down a tourist in a car, who took him to the park ranger station to get help. Chief Ranger Robert Peterson led the recovery team up the trail to Upper Emerald Pool, but they knew what they would find there. They managed to bring out Casalou's body by 3:00 p.m.

IN THE BLINK OF AN EYE

Norman Chin, a fifty-four-year-old geologist from Fullerton, California, came to Zion on his own in September 1969 and chose to hike the East Rim Trail on a pleasant Monday, September 22. No one saw him fall, but someone—presumably a family member—alerted rangers that he had gone missing. Three days later, on September 25, his body was spotted 1,200 feet below on the floor of the canyon. The best guess anyone can offer is that Chin slipped and fell while taking photographs of the astonishing rock formations around him.

When Steven Lee Miller fell from a cliff in the park on August 9, 1973, the incident also passed quietly and without fanfare. Miller, a native of Louisville, Kentucky, was camping in the park when he fell—and the media did not even note the location of the accident.

Details are equally vague for a twenty-year-old Idaho State University geology student named David Bourne, who camped with two friends at a backcountry site in the park with what district ranger Tony Bonanno described to the Associated Press as "a very exposed rim." Bourne fell to his death, probably in the middle of the night on March 16, 1978, tumbling 180 feet until he landed on a ledge. Whether he left the camp to relieve himself, rolled over the ledge in his sleep, or actually went wandering in the dark are unknown, but the medical examiner in Salt Lake City determined that Bourne died between midnight and 10:00 a.m. that morning. His two companions discovered that he was missing and peered over the cliff, spotting his body far below.

"In terms of recovery, it's fortunate he landed where he did—on a ledge," Bonanno continued. Otherwise, recovery of his body might have been impossible in the inaccessible canyon country far below the campsite.

In the case of Thomas Brereton, author of the book *Exploring the Backcountry of Zion National Park: Off-Trail Routes*, death came to the forty-two-year-old veteran hiker as a case of grave misfortune. He was hiking the southwest side of the West Temple (some accounts say Mount Kinesava) on April 13, 1979, when the rocks on which he was standing simply fell out from under him. He plummeted with the falling rocks. Some experienced hikers in this area believe that he stood on wet sandstone, which will crumble when saturated.

Nineteen-year-old John Russell, a student at Dixie College, intended to traverse the edge of a cliff at Middle Emerald Pool on October 16, 1983, when he stumbled and fell ninety feet into the gorge. Park rangers and a doctor were on the scene in short order, but they could do nothing for the young man.

In another example of sheer bad luck, thirty-five-year-old Larry Price of Crested Butte, Colorado, and his longtime friend Lawrence Rowlands climbed to the top of Court of the Patriarchs on November 22, 1994, but ran out of daylight before they could make it back to the trailhead. Price took a wrong step at about 8:00 p.m., missed the trail, and fell an estimated one hundred feet to his death. The search and recovery team brought his body out of the canyon the following day. "Preliminary findings indicate that not completing the climb in daylight may have contributed to his accident," the park's press release said.

Many years later, a second's lapse in attention resulted in the death of a park employee. On July 20, 2013, twenty-two-year-old Scott Schena, originally from Lowell, Massachusetts, spent a precious Saturday afternoon off from his job with Xanterra, the park's hospitality concessionaire, socializing with several other employees at Employee Falls, a watercourse behind the Zion Lodge employee housing area. When four other employees arrived to practice rappelling skills, he joined them and climbed above the falls. He walked near the edge at the top of the falls to wave to the group below, and in an instant he lost his footing and fell fifty feet onto the rocks below.

"Ranger/medics provided ALS medical care while evacuating Schena from the canyon," the next day's Zion morning report read. "During the evacuation, he became unresponsive and stopped breathing. Schena was resuscitated by the rangers and Lifeflight personnel and transported by air to Dixie Regional Medical Center, where he passed away."

Schena had worked the previous season in the Mt. McKinley Lodge at Denali National Park, and had planned a life of cooking and adventure travel work.

ALONE IN ZION

Few yearnings take on the awesome power of a solo hike in the wilderness, an exploration of the backcountry with nothing but your hiking skill, a few choice pieces of equipment, a pack full of food and supplies, and your wits. The opportunity to move at your own pace, linger where you wish, and wrap yourself in solitude can be so attractive that it pushes all thoughts of the potential dangers out of your consciousness. To wander like Thoreau or Whitman, to hear yourself think and to truly experience unbroken silence . . . what could be more appealing? Ah, wilderness!

Most people who attempt extended solo hikes probably come home unscathed, but we do not hear about those fortunate souls in the media. Instead, we hear the stories of the few who do not survive: Yi Jien Wa, who walked out into the Glacier National Park backcountry and vanished until bits of his remains were found four years later; Geraldine Largay, who left the Appalachian Trail to relieve herself and disappeared for two years, finally found dead of exposure in her tent in the Maine woods; Marie Caseiro, hiking near the Alta Ski Resort in Utah, who fell from a hundred-foot cliff off of a ski run in Little Cottonwood Canyon . . . and Affin William Phillips, a student at the University of Utah, who walked off into the Kolob section of Zion National Park with no climbing gear and no identification and did not come back alive.

"On the evening of May 14 [1993], two hikers advised the park that they had seen what they suspected were human remains in the rugged eastern end of the South Fork of Taylor Creek," the national park's morning report for May 1993 tells us. Mid-May remains a snowy, icy time in Zion's high country, so the first search party to attempt to locate these remains had to turn back to wait for daylight and to acquire more extensive gear. The following day, the Zion search and rescue team included climbing rangers and other local expert climbers, and their long search for the unidentified body finally ended after seven hours of "travel over extremely hazardous terrain, including ice bridges, precipitous snow-covered cliffs, and unstable ground."

The search and rescue team had hoped to use a helicopter to remove the body from the treacherous terrain, but the narrow canyon and the height of the surrounding cliffs made this impossible. Instead, the team worked together to move the body to a less remote and lower location. There they met the Washington County sheriff's rescue team, who assisted in hand-carrying the body back to the trailhead. "A total of ten people from three agencies were involved," the report said.

With no driver's license or other documents on the victim, the sheriff's office had to find some way to identify the body. After a fall of as much as one thousand feet, the body had sustained massive trauma, so immediate identification proved to be impossible—but the state medical examiner in Salt Lake City had more resources and was able to help. Luckily, one clue did turn up quickly: a lone car parked at the trailhead, a find that gave the sheriff a family to contact to see if the car's owner was missing. The family helped the medical examiner obtain dental records, leading him to identify the victim as twenty-one-year-old Phillips.

"The coroner ruled that Williams [*sic*] had died within 36 hours of the discovery of his body," the park report concluded. Sergeant Rymal Hinton of the Washington County Sheriff's Office told reporters at the Associated Press that it looked like Phillips had fallen because of the ice on the slopes. "He had neither climbing gear nor ropes and wore only sweat pants and moccasins," the wire service noted.

Not all hikers intend to be on their own in the back-country, but the decision to leave a larger group to double back to the trailhead can lead to unforeseen dangers. On May 16, 2001, Penny Lewis, a thirty-seven-year-old woman most recently from Beaumont, Texas, left her two companions in the Left Fork of North Creek (the trail also known as the Subway) to make her way back to the trailhead alone. Lewis had coached basketball at the University of Texas at Arlington, the University of Pacifica, and Quincy University in her hometown in Illinois; had served as assistant coach for the 1994 US Olympic Festival team; and had most recently become an assistant coach at the Division 1 level at Lamar University—so she had the athleticism and stamina to handle some rough trail hiking. Whether she had the specific skills needed to stay safe on a trail as demanding as the Subway is hard to say in retrospect. This permit-required hike involves wading through streams that are icy cold in mid-May, and climbing up steep slopes on uneven ground.

No one knows exactly what happened next, but some time later, two hikers found her "motionless and unresponsive on the trail," according to the park's morning report on the incident. Lewis was about a mile from the trailhead.

One of these hikers ran to the trailhead, flagged down a visitor in a car, explained the situation, and asked for a cell phone to call for help. The dispatch operator quickly reached a group of backcountry rangers on a training exercise fairly close to the trailhead, so they responded at once and reached Lewis quickly, where the other hiker had stayed with her. "They found that Lewis had no vital signs and that she'd been in that condition for at least 40 minutes," the report reads.

As protocol dictates, the rangers contacted Dixie Regional Medical Center and were advised not to attempt resuscitation, given that so much time had elapsed with no vital signs.

Investigators determined that Lewis had strayed from the trail and found herself at a high spot along the river, and that she attempted to work her way back to the trail down a long slope. "She apparently fell about 50 feet," the report concluded. Washington County sheriff Kirk Smith told the *Deseret News*, "There was some indication that she had fallen, but there was no apparent massive injury."

SLICKROCK IN HIDDEN CANYON

Some Zion hikes offer two kinds of experiences: a carefully planned trail for casual hikers with the reward of a magnificent view, and a more adventurous route beyond for people who enjoy a technical climb or a scramble. Hidden Canyon is just such a hike. It begins at the Weeping Rock trailhead, where many visitors head on their first day in the park to begin to adjust to the park's elevation with a short hike, and serpentines along the east side of the main canyon on a paved path. The trail then follows a series of switchbacks (no longer paved) to snake along the canyon wall, with some chains to provide a handhold. Finally, after a short descent, it climbs once again, this time up a series of steps chiseled out of stone. The trail ends with a walk along a narrow ledge to the beginning of the canyon, where you can enjoy the view of dark sandstone walls before either turning back—as most people do—or continuing into the canyon itself.

Those who choose to go on are in for a series of scrambles over boulders and slickrock, wanderings through more open areas, and the potential for some climbing. That's where twenty-seven-year-old Shawn Tuell ran into trouble while scrambling over slickrock with his uncle on August 1, 1998. Tuell simply slipped and fell, tumbling thirty feet and hitting his head on the way down. Remarkably, he survived the initial fall—but it took his uncle an hour and a half to hike out of the canyon and notify rangers that his nephew needed help.

Even with the gap in response time, however, Tuell still hung on until rescue crews reached him. They began life support, but Tuell went into cardiac arrest—and after an hour of CPR while waiting for a rescue helicopter to arrive from Nellis Air Force Base in Las Vegas, Tuell finally breathed his last. "More than twenty-five people were involved in the rescue, which ended at midnight," the *Deseret News* reported three days later.

WITNESS TO A FALL

Many national parks in the southern half of the country become centers of bustling activity on the day after Thanksgiving. Vacationers, local families, and others who have the rare Friday off come to the parks to begin to work off the previous day's feasting, making the most of the last days before the snows of winter render park roads and trails impassable.

On just such a day in 2008, Craig Forster, director of the University of Utah's Office of Sustainability, joined friends at Zion to launch the holiday season with a wilderness hike. They chose a trail through an unnamed canyon near Utah Route 9, and they had just scrambled up to a flat ledge at about 3:00 p.m. when the trail led them down a short slope. In the space of an instant, Forster lost his footing and slid down the slope to its end at a cliff edge. He managed to grip the edge and hang on for a moment, but not long enough for his friends to attempt a rescue—momentum forced him to let go and fall about twenty feet. His friends reached him in seconds and began CPR.

Others in the canyon saw him plunge off the edge, and one witness ran for help, notifying the rangers at the park's east entrance that "a man had fallen about twenty feet, landed mainly on his head and was unconscious when he [the witness] had left to get help," the park's news release stated. Rangers were on the scene within twelve minutes with an automated external defibrillator and a LIFEPAK defibrillator/monitor, and they used all of their capabilities to revive Forster. In the end, they were not successful.

A professor of hydrogeology in the university's architecture and planning department, Forster took on leadership of the Office of Sustainability because it was a student initiative—and he was never happier than when he was working with students, his wife, Bonnie Baty, told the *Deseret News* a few days after his death. "He liked the idea he was passing on the torch," she said. "Motivating people was one of his great loves."

Patrick Reimherr, president of the Associated Students of the University of Utah, echoed this observation. "It is rare when a professor will take a student project and help it come to life," he told the paper. "He incorporated students into the office well, he let students generate their own projects and worked with them to create success." Under Forster's leadership the office helped introduce sustainability solutions on campus, including a recycling program, installation of an efficient watering system, a campus farmer's market, and a cogeneration plant.

In Forster's honor, Utah State University—where he had been a faculty member in the geology department—established the Summit Fund, both to provide scholarships to geology students and to fund the annual Craig Forster Lecture Series, which presents topics of interest to geology students and scientists.

FAMILY TRAGEDY AT MIDDLE EMERALD POOL

Minutes before Tyler Jeffrey Eggertz slipped on a rock, his father, Jeffrey Eggertz, cautioned him and his sister, Brittany, to stay away from the ledge.

Tyler, who was twelve, hiked the Emerald Pools trail with his fifteen-year-old sister and a fourteen-year-old cousin. The three broke away from their father and the rest of the family at a fork in the trail and headed up the right branch from the Lower to the Middle Emerald Pool while the family took the left branch. Tyler and Brittany passed signs that informed them, "All three Emerald Pools and connecting creeks are closed to swimming, bathing and wading," and others that cautioned, "Stay on trail. Caution. Near the edge footing can be dangerous." Any parent can tell you, however, that teenagers pay little if any heed to such warnings.

When they reached the Middle Emerald Pool, the three children left the trail. They spotted a sandstone plateau they could use as a seat a short distance off the trail, about fifteen feet from the ledge, and sat there to dangle their feet into a side stream that terminated in a brisk cascade. The stream dropped over the nearby ledge.

One account says that Tyler simply tried to stand up, but a court document reports that he actually attempted to cross the stream. Whichever is more accurate, the result was the same: Tyler stepped on an algae-covered rock and his foot went out from under him. He fell into the stream, where the water was only about five inches deep, but it flowed strongly enough to drag him forward, out of his sister's reach, and pull him over the ledge. He plummeted one hundred feet, missed the plunge pool at the bottom of the falls, and instead hit the boulder garden next to it.

This all took place in the space of two or three heartbeats at 3:45 p.m. on March 28, 1997, in front of crowds of fellow hikers. Some attempted to provide first aid and revive the boy, but Tyler was pronounced dead at the scene.

Later, park spokesman Denny Davies told the *Deseret News* that had Brittany and the cousin tried to grab Tyler when he slipped, "They too would have fallen."

The story has a further bleak twist—Jeffrey Eggertz, his wife, Lora, and their three- and seven-year-old children had gone on another half mile to Upper Emerald Pool. They had lost sight of Tyler and Brittany, and expected to meet up with them again on the way down. Instead, they met a park ranger, who told them there had been a fatality at the middle pool.

"I asked if the family was with the person," Jeffrey said. He described his son to the ranger. In an instant of terrible clarity, he knew the boy in the accident was Tyler.

"You kind of go numb for a while, then it hits you," he told the *Deseret News*.

Tyler's mother, Nancy Elder, with whom Tyler lived in Sandy, described her son as an energetic boy whose passions included motorcycling, Scouting, rollerblading, and snowboarding. "He probably lived more in his twelve years than us if we lived to be one hundred," she told the *Deseret News*.

Tyler's death became a catalyst for some changes along the Emerald Pools trail. At the beginning of the trail, the park has added a sign that states, "Please: Watch your children—there are steep drop-offs. Swimming or wading in the pools is prohibited." A rope chain was installed near the Middle Emerald Pool to better define the path of the trail, and to discourage people from wandering off of it. The park moved some of the existing signs to make them more prominent. None of the signs specifically mentioned that rocks might become slippery with algae, however—and in February 2000, Jeffrey Eggertz and Nancy Elder filed a lawsuit against the United States of America, seeking $3.5 million in damages for the wrongful death of their son. Attorney Kathryn Collard, who represented the family in this case, told an Associated Press reporter, "I've always been of the mind that once you're in the woods, you are on your own. But this case has changed my mind."

The district court that heard the case ruled against the plaintiffs, and the parents brought the case to the US Court of Appeals for the Tenth Circuit. The judges affirmed the district court's decision in the case. "Plaintiffs challenge the adequacy of the signage existing at the time of the accident, including the two signs that said, 'Danger-Cliff. Slippery

Sandstone. Unstable Rock Edge. Wet Rock Hazardous,'" Judge Ruggero J. Aldisert wrote in his decision.

> *But what would constitute an adequate warning: Bigger signs? Signs embedded in the sandstone immediately next to each stream? Such "solutions," however, have an impact on park aesthetics. And even if Plaintiffs are contending only that the wording of existing signs should have been altered to mention algae specifically, such a change would necessitate a chain of further decisions. Would not Zion managers then have to decide whether it is necessary to add signs that explain how to identify algae . . . or that warn of the hazards of wet rock not covered by algae, and whether such additional signage would impair the scenery too much, as well as numb visitors to all warnings?*

The judge's assessment of the problem states exactly the kind of decisions every national park faces on a daily basis. In the end, this case and all the others in this book serve as fair warnings to park visitors: Every trail, every climb, and every river and stream can be hazardous. National parks push us to take personal responsibility for every step we take—and when we let our guard slip, an accident can lead to a tragedy.

CHAPTER 5

Daring Fate: Climbing, Canyoneering, and BASE Jumping Accidents

A QUICK WORD: I'VE SEPARATED THE LIST OF EIGHTEEN deaths in Zion resulting from climbing, canyoneering, and BASE jumping from other kinds of falls in the park because these incidents involve a different set of skills and more significant risk. Technical climbing, scaling a sheer rock face, rappelling down a canyon wall, and actually jumping out into clear air stand out from the hiker who loses his or her footing and slips over the edge of a cliff. I am not a climber or canyoneer, so I will make no attempt to determine why these unlucky souls fell; if you want to participate in such discussions, plenty of websites speculate on the most recent of these cases.

꩜

On the day that Don Orcutt became the first man to successfully climb the Great White Throne, he discovered that someone had been there before him.

There atop the 6,744-foot white Navajo sandstone monolith on June 30, 1931, Orcutt found "a portion of a human skull, yellow and brittle with age," the *Iron County Record* reported several weeks later. "In years gone by some unknown climber has scaled the cliffs of the Great White Throne in the park, but never returned to report the exploit."

With no other information on the hapless climber, the newspaper was left to speculate on the origin of the human artifact. "Perhaps in days forgotten some venturesome Indian, perhaps of the cliff dwelling nation, made his way to the top, but after reaching there feared to make the descent and remained, awaiting the rescue party which never came."

It's as likely a story as any, as this skull is the only clue we have about a person who perished in what would become Zion National Park, probably hundreds of years before a system of national parks was ever conceived. We do know quite a bit about the man who found the artifact, however—and about the infamy he achieved not only for being the first to climb the Great White Throne, but for the fate that befell him shortly thereafter.

A seasoned climbing veteran with uncommon experience and skill, twenty-four-year-old Orcutt scaled Mount Whitney—at the time the highest mountain in the United States, as Alaska was not yet a state, so Mt. Denali did not count as the country's highest peak—as well as Mount Hood, Mount Rainier, and many other peaks in the High Sierras. His climb of the Great White Throne began at the floor of the canyon at 6:00 a.m. on June 30, and by 10:30 a.m. he signaled from the top that he had summited the peak successfully. "He is reported to have named this the hardest climb he had ever made," the *Iron County Record* noted.

The legendary climb was not without mishap. "Orcutt, who climbed barefoot"—yes, barefoot—"slipped once and slid 40 or 50 feet toward certain death," the *Garfield County News* reported. "He stopped just before it was too late. Hugging a rock, he finally made his way out of danger."

Perhaps this shoeless predilection contributed to what happened to Orcutt just one month later. On July 28, 1931, he decided to climb another of Zion's peaks, this one considered "not very dangerous" to seasoned climbers. He planned to scale Cathedral Mountain, making it a practice run before he attempted another first later in the summer: West Temple Mountain. No human being had summited West Temple at that point, so Orcutt set his sights on it.

He left the canyon at 11:00 a.m. to begin his Cathedral ascent—and while climbing enthusiasts doubtless will want to know exactly which route he took up the mountain, this information does not appear in the reports available. What we do know is that he ascended the mountain by "easy stages," and when he failed to return by late in the afternoon, park rangers knew that something had gone wrong.

They soon found the badly mangled body of Don Orcutt about a mile and a half from the West Rim Trail. "Rangers estimated that he had fallen about 1,000 feet over the jagged slopes of the mountain," the *Iron County Record* said. "His body was mangled almost beyond recognition when found."

Even in death, Orcutt managed to secure one more first for his permanent record: He was the first climber to die in

Zion National Park, and only the second visitor to the park to die there as well (the story of the first, Albin Brooksby, is in chapter 9).

A Step Too Far, a Jolt Too Sudden

After Don Orcutt's death, thirty-four years passed before another climber met his end at Zion—and this time, he had a close connection to the park. He was fifteen-year-old Ronald Hillery, the son of Allen R. Hillery, Zion park roads and trails foreman.

On October 10, 1965, at about 1:00 p.m., Ron and his friend Steve Anderson, who was sixteen, were climbing at a small waterfall in Lodge Canyon behind the employee housing area, an activity that had kept the two boys and a group of friends busy on and off for several days. Anderson said that he and Ron were trying to retrieve a climbing piton and a rope from a ledge. "Ron had climbed up to unfasten the role from the peton [sic]," Anderson told the Associated Press. "He leaned out from the ledge . . . and the next thing I heard him scream 'Steve' and he fell."

Ron fell thirty feet, landing on his head among the rocks. He died two hours later in a St. George hospital of massive internal injuries.

It was 1992 before another climber perished in the park. David Faulkner Bryant, an assistant attorney general for the State of Utah, planned a day of canyoneering on October 10 with two friends in the Subway portion of North Creek. The group tied their rope to a small pinion pine tree on the edge of the canyon, and Bryant was the last to rappel down the canyon wall at about 3:15 p.m. On the way, however, he slipped briefly and caught himself with the rope, and the shock to the line pulled the tree out of the ground by the roots. Bryant fell backward about thirty feet and landed hard on the rocks below.

More than a dozen other climbers and hikers witnessed his fall, including a doctor who rushed to Bryant's side. He quickly determined that Bryant was not breathing, but he had a pulse, so the doctor went to work to attempt to save him. The doctor used the handle of a plastic milk bottle to create an airway and intubated the unfortunate man, beginning ventilations as one of Bryant's companions hiked out of the Subway to get help.

Given the remoteness of the Subway, it took the hiker more than an hour to reach a phone to call 911. Park rangers received the dispatch call at 4:45 p.m. and immediately contacted Nellis Air Force Base to request a helicopter. Nearly four hours later, at 8:30 p.m., Bryant finally arrived at a hospital in St. George, but his injuries were too severe to survive. He passed away shortly thereafter.

Five more years passed before another climber made a fatal error in Zion. This time, it was John Christensen's fall off of Angels Landing, a story told in chapter 3.

Deadly Adventures

The origins of canyoneering in Utah—exploring canyons by hiking, wading, swimming, rock climbing, and rappelling—stretch back to the days of the Anasazi people, with European-descended explorers accelerating the pace in the 1800s as they "discovered" the canyon lands in this territory. Not until the mid- to late twentieth century did it become a popular sport with the most adventurous visitors to Zion and other canyon parks and recreation areas. With advances in the safety, usability, and availability of the required technical gear and the explosion of information made available online, the sport's popularity accelerated . . . and with it, the number of fatalities in Zion grew.

Some of these came about through nothing more than bad luck, a person standing in the wrong place at precisely the right time. Twenty-year-old Sasha Simpson, for example, died in January 1999 while standing still. She was waiting on a ledge on the Mountain of the Sun mountaineering route, near the end of the route at Falling Water Hanging Garden Cliffs, while another in her party freed a rope that was stuck in a crevice. Suddenly a rock gave way above her. She swerved to avoid being hit by the rock and lost her balance, tumbling 150 feet down the cliff face and sustaining fatal head injuries.

Even highly skilled canyoneers can find themselves in deadly trouble. On September 6, 2003, rescue teams at Zion faced the chilling task of bringing a friend out of the park after he fell from a wall in Behunin Canyon. Christopher Frankewicz of Springdale, an experienced and skilled climber and canyoneer, attempted a one-day descent through the canyon—a task that normally takes about eight hours, according to the park's morning report the following day. When friends reported to rangers that he had not returned by the evening of September 5, a search and rescue team set out early the following morning to find him. "Frankewicz's body was found just after noon at the base of one of the rappels in the middle of the canyon," the report said. "It appears that he fell 60 to 80 feet while attempting to locate the rappel station."

In the case of Roselan "Ross" Tamin, a thirty-five-year-old visitor from Bournemouth, England, traveling with his lifelong friend Richard Connors, the accident that ended his life on May 21, 2002, came about because of a knot that did not hold.

The two had been on the road in the United States for several weeks, exploring a number of national parks and other points of interest, and they planned a climb of the Spaceshot, "an area popular for rappelling in the park," according to the *Spectrum*, the St. George newspaper. Spaceshot is on the east side of Zion Canyon, between the Temple of Sinawava and Big Bend, not far from the road. The two men cut their climb short when they noticed storm clouds forming, deciding instead to rappel back to the bottom.

"The two were on the face of the mountain when apparently the ropes of the victim's line failed," said Washington County sheriff Kirk Smith to *Spectrum* reporter Patrice St. Germain. "There was a boulder in between the two and the friend heard the victim scream and by the time he got past the boulder, he saw his partner was gone."

Tamin fell about 180 feet to the rocky surface below.

Another visitor heard Connors yelling for help, flagged down a shuttle bus driver, and told the driver to call for emergency assistance. "Dispatch received the call for help at approximately 10 a.m.," the *Spectrum* said. "Park rangers were dispatched to the scene and found Tamin with no detectable signs of life."

What exactly had happened to Tamin remained a mystery to the many canyoneering enthusiasts across the country who heard about the accident. Had his rope actually failed in some catastrophic way? Had one of the two men bungled a knot? What innocent mistake had the visitors from England made—and how could other climbers avoid making the same error?

After weeks of speculation on canyoneering newsgroups and discussion boards, Connors himself demonstrated an uncommon generosity to the global canyoneering community by posting on June 14, 2002, a detailed account of the steps that led up to his friend's death, on the uk.rec.climbing newsgroup. (Connors uses the word *abseil*, which is another word for *rappel*.)

I got to the top of pitch 4 as Ross arrived at the top of pitch 3. Ross had got some two-way radios earlier on the trip and we chatted on the radio: the weather forecast had been slowly deteriorating for the last 3 days, today was 50% chance of afternoon rain, there were a lot of gloomy clouds brewing above us, the sandstone is all bad in the wet, we were not super fast aid climbers . . . A brief spot of rain actually hit us and we decided to bail. I pulled up the 9mm rope, tied it to the yellow, stripped the anchor and descended to the top of pitch 3. Meantime Ross had been untying the green from this anchor and getting ready to set up a double-rope abseil. I got down to him, chucked him the end of the yellow to tie to the green and started pulling the ropes down from above.

Ross headed off down to the big sandy ledge as I coiled the 9mm and put it on my back. He radioed me to say "rope free" and I headed down. I arrived on the big sandy ledge about 10–15ft away from the anchor—Ross was off to my left, already clipped into the anchor and sorting out the blue rope, ready to set up the last abseil. I chucked the loose end of the yellow to Ross and started pulling the ropes from above. I was unclipped at this point—being a very bad boy, even though it was a huge ledge. This was actually the only thing that struck me as unsafe about our whole day. As the knot came down, I stopped and untied it to free the yellow, which was now all tangled up in plants and rocks on the ledge. Ross fed it over the edge as I untangled it from everything on the ledge. I started pulling the green down as Ross sorted himself out over at the anchor. I was coiling the green rope as Ross called over to say "see you at the bottom in a few minutes," he saw me coiling the green and offered to carry it, since I had the 9mm already on my back, but he already had our daysack on so I said I was fine taking it down. I turned to just finish up coiling the green and at that moment he fell.

I rushed over and there was nothing there—our ropes had gone, Ross had gone, the anchor was fine, untouched. Everything floated for a moment, slipped sideways and turned unreal—then I started shouting . . . I knew I had to get down in case by some impossible chance there was something I could do to help him. I was yelling down to the road and got someone's attention, they flagged down one of the shuttle buses and shouted that help was coming. I had the 55m green and the 50mx9mm ropes with me. I couldn't get to the ground in one go but I knew there was another anchor (top of the Alpine Start for those that know it) that I would be able to reach. I set up the double rope abseil and set off down. The ropes tangled around everything—it was a complete shambles. I saw the rangers and the ambulance arrive; the rangers were racing up the hill to Ross. I set up the second abseil, it was all taking so long . . . as I reached the ground one of the rangers came over to tell me what I already knew.

Some stuff that I do know—Ross was found with the two ropes correctly through his belay device. The ropes extended about 10 feet "above" him (the other 190 feet being "below" his belay device) and the ends were not tied together. Throughout this trip we had always been tying ropes together using a fig-eight knot . . . The only other abseil Ross set up that same day (from top of pitch 3 down to the big ledge) he had used the fig-eight knot with no back up knot on the tails. The knot was neat, I don't remember exactly how long the tails were but they didn't cause me a second glance. I could not see exactly what Ross was setting up on that last abseil—he was 10 ft or so to my left and was sitting (while clipped in) so that he obscured my view of the anchor.

The important bit—Some guys that were helping me out played around in their yard with this fig-eight method, tying it and trying to pull the knot apart. They found some worrying things. The way the ropes pull on this knot on a double-rope abseil deforms the knot badly.

If the knot is not perfectly "dressed," in particular if there is a single slack loop anywhere on the fig-eight, they could pull the knot through even with 6 INCHES of tails, just pulling the ropes apart as happens naturally on an abseil. 6 inches of tails is NOT ENOUGH. If you use this knot, tie a back up knot and leave LONG tails. It scares me to think that I could have innocently/ignorantly made this same catastrophic mistake.

Connors went on to express his sorrow at losing his friend, and added, "The only other thing I want to say here is that the rangers at Zion were incredible; the way they dealt with the incident, the diligence of their investigation and the compassion that they showed me . . . I have only praise for everything they did. I was overwhelmed by the generosity of so many other people in Springdale—it's a small town of wonderful people. Despite everything, I have some very fond memories of Zion and the people I met. It is a beautiful place—you should go there and climb those amazing walls."

DEATH BY TECHNICALITY

Canyoneering and climbing are highly technical sports, activities in which participants wager their lives against their own ability to rig their equipment properly. Most accidents—at least in Zion—take place not because the equipment itself failed, but because of a second's worth of slip-up, a rope run through an incorrectly blocked carabiner or a knot that lacks enough tail for safety under load. Sometimes canyoneers run out of daylight before they finish a route, working in the dark to make the last descent. Others simply fall off a ledge.

At forty-eight years old, Keith Biedermann of Garden Grove, California, had climbed up and rappelled down many walls, often in the company of others who shared his love of the experience. "I've been told [Biedermann] was a dedicated and serious hiker or mountaineer type," Lieutenant Jake Adams of the Washington County Sheriff's Office told reporter Ryan Hammill at the *Orange County Register*.

On June 4, 2007, Biedermann and two friends obtained the proper permit to explore Heaps Canyon, a popular canyoneering route near Emerald Pools, described by Tom Jones in his online Utah Canyoneering Guide as "a truly wonderful canyon, but it is also BIG. Deep inside the mountain, it is dark, wet, sinuous, and moody . . . Heaps saves the best for last—a series of raps culminating in a 280-foot free-hanging the whole way rappel, with the wall at least 50 feet away. AWESOME, and something you want to be alert for."

At the end of a day of exploring the canyon, Biedermann and his friends began the lengthy process of making the final 280-foot rappel. The first two went down carefully and landed without any serious mishaps. Biedermann began his rappel with a companion holding the belaying rope as he descended . . . and the rope suddenly went slack. Biedermann fell the remaining 260 feet to his death.

Over the course of the investigation, rangers and Biedermann's companions put together a working theory of the accident's cause, one involving the connection at the top of the rope (the "locking biner") slipping through the carabiner that was supposed to hold it in place. The deadly rappel took place between 10:30 and 11:00 p.m., and while the men all had headlamps, the combination of fatigue, darkness, and trepidation about making the long, free-hanging descent all certainly could have contributed to the error that ended Biedermann's life.

An equipment issue contributed to the death of thirty-four-year-old James Martin Welton on October 17, 2008, during his ascent of Touchstone, a thousand-foot wall across the canyon from Angels Landing. Welton, who came from Durango, Colorado, had climbed El Capitan in Yosemite National Park earlier that year, and his friends, family, and fellow climbers considered him an experienced climber with advanced skills. On this fall evening in Zion, he and two friends—Matt Tuttle of Kamas, Utah, and Robert Hooker of Elko, Nevada—had made it up the first three hundred feet of the climb and expected to spend the night on the cliff face on port-a-ledges—cots attached to the rock wall some distance above them.

Welton was climbing a rope using a mechanical ascender (also called a jumar), according to the park's morning report the day after the accident. This device slides freely in one direction—up the rope—and stops by gripping the rope when pulled in the opposite direction. The climber attaches the ascender to his or her harness before clipping it onto the rope, and then deploys the device's locking mechanism to keep it from sliding off the end of the rope.

"Preliminary investigation reveals that Welton was climbing a rope using mechanical ascenders," the morning report said. "It appears that a short fall occurred, causing the ascenders to sever the rope."

A National Park Service news release provided additional information: "It appears the ascenders may not have been fully engaged, resulting in a 20-foot fall along the rope. When the ascenders did fully engage, the shock severed the rope."

As his friends looked on helplessly from other points on the wall, Welton fell three hundred feet to his death.

Two other climbers ascending a different route nearby managed to flag down one of the park buses and report the accident. When the eleven-member search and rescue team arrived, however, the mission quickly became one of recovery of Welton's body and investigation of the incident. The team worked through the night to determine what had made a known climbing expert—one who also worked as a mountain first responder—die in a precipitous drop off the rock face.

A member of the investigation team posted a lengthy description of what happened on the climbing site Super-Topo, including this fairly straightforward summation that will make sense to people with climbing experience: "James somehow malfunctioned the attachment of his jumars to the taught haul line, but after he had released his daisy chains from the anchor. He began sliding down the haul line until one of his jumars finally engaged some 30 feet later or so. There was a sheath piling found on the scene, so we know he broke the sheath first, initiated a sheath fall, and finally the core broke after the sheath fall ended and shock-loaded the system. He and the bags fell 300 feet to the base."

THE DANGERS OF INEXPERIENCE

Hiking the Subway, also known as the Left Fork of North Creek, requires more than a little skill in route finding, crossing and recrossing the creek, finding a way around or over large boulders, and—depending on which route you take— swimming across deep pools of water just barely above the freezing point. "Visitors are encouraged to do the trip with an experienced hiker of The Subway, or obtain a detailed route description," the park's website tells us. Whether hikers choose to start at the Left Fork trailhead on Kolob Terrace Road and work their way up the canyon, or start at the top at the Wildcat Canyon trailhead and follow the complex route down, the Subway provides a nine-plus-mile daylong adventure for the most intrepid canyoneers—and a potential disaster for those who have little idea what lies ahead.

That being said, this hike has become so popular that the park limits the number of hikers to eighty per day, distributing permits by lottery before opening reservations for whatever scant spaces remain. Visitors who brave this route discover a world of knife-slice slot canyons, tunnels, twists, deep blue pools, and polished rock formations that make the struggle to see them seem that much more worth doing.

The words *strenuous* and *beginner canyoneering* are both used by Utah hiking websites to describe this route, seemingly contradictory terms that make it difficult to know what to expect. The top-down route involves several short rappels, roughly fifteen feet each, some of which lead down waterfalls—but with the hardware already in place along the route, these may make people new to canyoneering feel more confident about their skills than may be wise. This is the frame of mind that led Yoshio Hosobuchi, a seventy-four-year-old neurosurgeon from Novato, California, and his sixty-one-year-old wife, Dresden, into the Subway to check off one more great adventure from his bucket list.

Challenge did not scare this couple. For one, Hosobuchi had performed uncounted numbers of complex brain surgeries in the course of his career, and there are pages of tributes to him from grateful patients in the annals of the Internet. The Hosobuchis had hiked Mount Kilimanjaro the previous year, and they took an introductory course in canyoneering when they arrived in Springdale and followed it with a hike in Keyhole Canyon, a route that involved three rappels to get into the slender slot canyon, earlier in the week. They had never been in the Subway, however, and were eager to see the natural formations secreted inside.

They began their hike in the canyon on the morning of September 18, 2012, and about midway into the canyon, they reached the top of a waterfall. Hosobuchi spotted an anchor in the falls and one on the opposite side, so rather than cross the creek to use the one farther off, he decided to rappel from the anchor in the water.

No sooner did he begin his descent than something went wrong. "His rappelling device jammed, possibly because of a knot," the *Salt Lake Tribune* reported three days later. His foot caught in the rope, and "he wound up upside down, his hands about five feet above the ground."

Other reports, including one in the *Great Falls Tribune*, suggest that the man chose this vertical descent over the gentler rock slab, leaving him "unable to use his feet to maintain traction with the rock."

Hosobuchi could not pull himself upright, nor could he reach his foot to free it. His wife had already climbed down to the base of the falls without rappelling. She did her best to reach the jammed device or to free his foot, but she did not succeed. "They were the last ones in the canyon, having been passed by several groups throughout the day," the *Salt Lake Tribune* said. The time was about 5:30 p.m.

There was only one thing left for her to do: Hike out of the canyon and try to get help. She left her husband dangling in the waterfall and headed down toward the far end of the route.

Here, however, is where the Hosobuchis may have grossly overestimated their own skills. With nothing more than an introductory class in wayfinding and no real-world experience, Dresden could not find her way out. "The partner was caught by darkness and was unfamiliar with the exit route, and could not make it out of the canyon," said Aly Baltrus, park spokesperson, to *Salt Lake Tribune* reporters Bob Mims and Michael McFall.

She made her way back to her husband and stayed with him until daylight, sitting essentially alone in the pitch-dark night.

Meanwhile, a canyoneer from one of the groups that had passed the Hosobuchis called park dispatch at about 9:00 p.m. He said that based on the pace at which the couple was moving when he saw them, they would not make it out of the canyon that night and would be forced to stay overnight. Rangers planned to leave on a search mission early the following morning to see what had happened to the older couple. They "ran into Hosobuchi's wife on the trail about 11:45 a.m. as she was hiking out," the *Tribune* reported.

An hour later, they found Hosobuchi himself, still hanging by one foot in the cold rushing water. He had passed away during the night.

The Associated Press interviewed hiking guide Mike Banach, who had a working familiarity with the Subway through his own experience. He explained that "hanging in a harness for too long, especially upside-down, can cut off a climber's blood circulation."

"The Subway is deceiving," park superintendent Jock Whitworth said in a park news release issued later that day. "It is a very popular trail, but very difficult ... Unfortunately, its location inside the wilderness also means that rescues are not always possible or timely enough. Sound decision making and problem solving are critical."

The search and recovery team had to wait another full day for a helicopter to remove Hosobuchi's body from the Subway. When a more thorough examination was possible, authorities determined that when the rope jammed in the belay device, Hosobuchi "used a knife to cut his waist belt in an effort to free himself," the *Deseret News* reported. "However, the harness slipped down his legs and became entangled with his right foot as he tumbled over head-first inside the waterfall. Hosobuchi appeared to be pinned by the force of the rushing water."

Baltrus offered a cautionary word to others who may consider taking on the Subway as their first major canyoneering outing. "Our message is you can learn the basics of canyoneering, but what happens when something goes wrong is hard to teach quickly," she said.

THE PACE QUICKENS

Since 2011 Zion has seen increases in the number of annual visitors who have discovered this magnificent park—from 2,847,403 visitors in 2011 to 4,317,028 in 2016. Perhaps this is the reason that the number of climbing, canyoneering, and (briefly) BASE jumping accidents in the park has increased as well. (More on BASE jumping later in this chapter.)

Just five weeks after Yoshio Hosobuchi's tragic accident, climber Lyle David Hurd III, age forty-nine, and three companions took on the Northeast Buttress route below Angels Landing, a first for Hurd—although he had climbed a number of other big walls in Zion and was considered an experienced and skilled climber. Traveling two by two with Hurd and his partner following the other pair, Hurd "was leading the fifth pitch when he fell over 40 feet onto a ledge, pulling his top piece of protection out," the park's news release informed readers. His climbing partner, Mark Engibous, saw him fall and immediately called 911; he was an intensive care unit nurse and started first aid, talking with Hurd—who was awake and alert at that point—as the other pair of climbers set up a top rope for the rescue team and waited for it to arrive. Three hours passed until the local team reached them, but despite the care Engibous gave him, Hurd could not hold out that long without more extensive medical assistance. The search and rescue team worked through the night to bring Hurd's body out of the park.

On September 5, 2013, forty-seven-year-old Cheri Haas and three friends set out on the approach path to the Subway for a challenging all-day hike. Haas was in the lead on the trail when she missed a hard right turn and continued straight and off the trail. Her boyfriend and two friends saw her vanish as she fell over a cliff.

While the friends ran for help, Haas's boyfriend rappelled down the cliff to find her. He discovered that she had not survived the hundred-foot fall—and also that it would be very difficult to bring her out of this part of the canyon. So rugged and forbidding was the terrain here that the park's search and rescue team contacted Grand Canyon National Park for a helicopter and crew. The job of recovering her body continued well into the next day.

Just three days before, visitor Clark Profitt had slipped over a cliff edge in Behunin Canyon and survived, most likely because he was wearing a helmet. The park's superintendent commented on both in a bulletin published by the *St. George News.* "In both instances, we strongly suspect that these events were caused by getting too close to the edge of a cliff," superintendent Jock Whitworth said. "Loose sand on slickrock may have been the cause of the falls. Given the topography of Zion National Park, these accidents could have occurred anywhere, even popular trails in the main canyon, including Angels Landing and Observation Point. All of us need to maintain situational awareness and be extremely careful anytime we are near an edge."

A year later, on October 19, 2014, forty-seven-year-old Christopher Spencer of San Jose, California, and a climbing partner were on an approach pitch on the Iron Messiah route—described by the park as "a technical 5.10 climb in Zion Canyon"—when Spencer fell backward. Had he been roped in, he may have been able to break his fall, or he may have pulled his partner with him on his eighty-foot tumble down the steep slope. Spencer struck a series of ledges on his way down, and the park's news release made specific reference to the fact that he was not wearing a helmet.

Rangers were dispatched at about 11:00 a.m. and reached Spencer in less than an hour along with a Lifeflight medical crew. The emergency medical technicians stabilized Spencer and kept him alive during the three-hour evacuation, but once he arrived at Dixie Regional Medical Center, he succumbed to his massive injuries.

In 2015 Zion saw a 34 percent increase in the number of emergency medical services (EMS) calls and a 56 percent increase in the number of searches and rescues required over the previous year. By July 6 the park had had 175 EMS calls and 57 search and rescue calls, often responding to more than one call per day. Between July 5 and 12, the park responded to 16 EMS calls. The volume of calls in the summer of 2015 gives testimony to the skills of these rescuers: Only one of these emergencies resulted in a loss of life.

On July 12, 2015, canyoneer Bryan Artmann, a twenty-four-year-old man from Henderson, Nevada, was on his first journey through Heaps Canyon, one of the most challenging canyons in the park, involving three thousand feet of descent. He had just completed a climb at about 7:00 p.m. and paused on top of a mesa to have a look around when something—only he could know what—went wrong in the course of a split second. He took an unroped, hundred-foot fall down the side of the mesa.

One of the men with him later posted to a discussion board that the accident occurred in "the 'keyhole' area after the iron room." Only those who have traversed the canyon will understand this, but I am including it for your reference.

Artmann's three companions had no choice but to descend down the mesa to reach him, and while one of them remained with him, the other two traversed the rest of the canyon at top speed to get help—a process that took until 11:30 p.m.

Once again, the Zion search and rescue team called in a helicopter from Grand Canyon to help make the recovery. Hoping that the mission would be a rescue instead of a recovery, two Zion team members were short-hauled into Heaps Canyon above the victim—that is, they were suspended below the helicopter for the fastest possible deployment—and rappelled down to reach him. They learned quickly that Artmann had passed away during the night. It took a total of sixteen search and rescue crewmembers to reach Artmann and remove his body from the canyon.

Three months of additional EMS calls and rescues continued through the summer and early fall. On October 2, 2015, Zion Dispatch alerted rangers that a satellite emergency notification device (SEND) had been activated in the vicinity of the technical canyoneering route in Imlay Canyon. Whoever had turned the device on proceeded to turn it on and off over the next several hours, reactivating it repeatedly in an effort to get the attention of rescue personnel.

Classic Helicopter, a local service, did an aerial search over the canyon to attempt to locate the group, and a ranger proceeded to the canyon's exit route area to attempt to gather information. At 2:15 p.m. two canyoneers reached the Grotto and reported that they had been with the party that set off the SEND. They had begun that morning to traverse Not Imlay Canyon, a side canyon of Imlay Canyon that had grown in popularity over the last several years. Not Imlay offered a shorter, drier route compared to Imlay Canyon, with a similar level of technical difficulty.

"Their group of four planned to rappel this canyon, when the first person on rappel fell and was not responsive to shouts from the canyon rim," a blog on the Zion National Park website noted. "A SEND device was activated immediately while two of the group members hiked out to the Grotto to report the incident. The third group member remained on scene with the SEND device."

Taking the helicopter to the canyon, rangers rappelled to the fallen individual, reaching him at 7:20 p.m. They discovered that he was Christian Louis Johnson, known locally as Louis—a fifty-year-old St. George resident who regularly explored Zion with his husband, Everett Boutillet. The rangers confirmed that Johnson had not survived the two-hundred-foot fall.

What had gone wrong for this skilled group? Something basic: Their rope was too short. Columnist Dallas Hyland of the St. George *Independent* had an extensive conversation with Boutillet about the incident, and shared this description with his readers:

Everett says the rope did not reach the first landing due to a recent change in the location of the second rappel station they were not aware of. Louis did not look in time to realize he was in trouble and by the time he knew, he was only able to shout up that the end of the rope was eight feet from the landing. He presumably had no choice but to try to land on his feet in a treacherous place as the rappel was multi-pitched. This means he would ideally have tied in to the second anchor before coming off the first rope but was unable to. The party could not see Louis but heard him come off the rope and land, and they believe he rolled off the second rappel unroped.

Boutillet added, "The sounds suggest this and will never leave my mind."

The tragedy of Johnson's death serves as a reminder to even the most experienced canyoneers and climbers that anyone—from a beginner on his or her first climb to an expert who routinely leads others—can make a miscalculation that can result in disaster. Johnson and Boutillet had "descended more than 100 canyons 200 times in five states," as Boutillet told the media on the day of the accident. "Zion was our favorite park. Our favorite place to be. Our first canyon was the 'Subway' and we were instantly addicted. Louis and I understood the risks, but the joy that it brought outweighed them."

EXPERIENCE IS NO GUARANTEE

The story in *Rock and Ice* magazine begins by calling Eric Michael Klimt "an accomplished climber and teacher." Klimt had enough confidence in his own abilities and in his familiarity with the route to take on Zion's Moonlight Buttress alone on March 9, 2016. He was planning on "rope-soloing the upper pitches by rappelling in from the top," his family told journalist Hayden Carpenter.

What exactly went wrong is still a matter of discussion on climbing websites, but at about 12:30 p.m., another group of climbers at the bottom of the route watched in horror as Klimt hurtled into the canyon in free fall. Park rangers recovered his body 1,200 feet below the summit. "He was found wearing an intact harness with a GriGri [assisted braking belay device] attached to his belay loop with a carabiner," Carpenter wrote. The GriGri, manufactured by Petzl, assists in braking under a shock load—if the climber suddenly drops a few feet, for example, it can stop him or her in the midst of a rapid descent. "The rest of his gear was still at the top of the climb."

Writers Chris Van Leuven and Corey Buhay could provide little additional insight in their article for the *Alpinist* as to what had made this thirty-six-year-old veteran climber and teacher suddenly topple from a rock face he knew well. "For the past several years, Klimt, originally from Baltimore, Maryland, had been practicing the free moves on Moonlight Buttress," they wrote, noting that this was one of the park's most popular big wall climbs. Klimt's two decades of experience extended to climbs in Yosemite National Park, Red Rock Canyon National Recreation Area, Joshua Tree National Park, and North Conway, New Hampshire. "On the morning of March 9 he rappelled on a single line onto the route's top pitches to work on free moves and gear placements. Sometime later something went wrong."

His brother, Carl, told Van Leuven and Buhay that Eric had tried this particular route—following a series of cracks in the Navajo sandstone—three times since 2013, but he struggled to link all the moves.

Information Van Leuven and Buhay gathered from the family and from Zion rangers did not fill in the blanks. "Zion National Park officials aren't certain which pitch he fell from," they noted. "Officials said his single rope was attached to the anchor with clove hitches on opposed carabiners. Two slings were around his torso, a few cams and nuts were on his harness, and his Grigri was clipped to his belay loop with a locking carabiner. The Grigri had no obvious damage, his 9.8mm 70m rope had no noticeable damage and his hands did not show signs of rope burn."

The only other clue: There was no knot tied on the bottom end of his rope. Experts finally came to the conclusion that Klimt had become detached from his self-belay system.

"He was not wearing a helmet," the *Alpinist* writers added, a refrain that had become common in twenty-first century stories of climbing accidents and deaths.

Klimt was working in Chattanooga, Tennessee, in the months before the accident, using his climbing skills in the inspection, maintenance, and construction industry as a rope access technician. Finding this not as stable a work situation as he needed, he planned to move to Terrebonne, Oregon, where he had lived the previous fall. He had uncommon skill as a high school math teacher as well. His brother Carl told the *Alpinist* writers, "He loved the beauty and symmetry of math [and] nature."

FOR A MOMENT OF FLIGHT

For Amber Bellows and her husband of two weeks, Clayton Butler, risky sports were central to their relationship.

They met at a skydiving facility in Tooele, Utah, in 2011, where Bellows had come to take her first course in jumping out of a plane. She and Butler dated for three years and married in late January 2014, completing their special day with a BASE jump: They leapt from their hotel room on the twenty-seventh floor of the MGM Signature in Las Vegas, opening parachutes almost immediately after stepping off the balcony into clear air. They landed safely (albeit dramatically) on a city street, as they had in all the jumps they had made over the previous three years.

Their luck ran out two weeks later.

A BASE jump is a leap from a stationary structure or object (the acronym stands for Building, Antenna, Span—such as a bridge—or Earth, including cliffs and peaks). A successful jump involves a brief, intensely thrilling free fall and an almost immediate deployment of a parachute—a critically important factor, because a BASE jumper is much closer to the ground than a skydiver, who has thousands of feet of air in which a parachute can inflate. Jumping from the balcony of a Las Vegas hotel room, for example, meant that Bellows and Butler were only three hundred feet or so off the ground, so their parachutes had to deploy and inflate in the first second or two of their fall.

On February 8, 2014, the newlyweds hiked to the top of Mount Kinesava—a strenuous four-and-a-half-mile trek to the top of the 7,276-foot peak, which may have taken the couple as long as nine hours—and prepared to make their jump off of the peak's east side. The position provided them with about two thousand feet for their free fall, giving them precious seconds of plummeting descent before they deployed their parachutes and floated safely to the canyon floor.

Bellows leaped first, and Butler followed an instant later. In seconds he knew that his wife's parachute had failed to open, but he could not reach her to attempt to save her. He saw her plunge into the rocky canyon.

Butler landed safely and had no choice but to hike out of the remote backcountry for help. It was 6:30 p.m. before he could notify park officials of the accident.

Park rangers knew that the mission to bring the twenty-eight-year-old woman out of the backcountry would be one of recovery rather than rescue, and that a helicopter would be required to locate her body. They contacted Grand Canyon National Park for use of the larger park's helicopter and crew, and flew over the backcountry at the base of Mount Kinesava to locate Bellows's body in the snow-covered canyon. Once they knew the extent of the challenges involved, they planned a short-haul operation—suspending two rangers beneath the helicopter until they reached the young woman, so they could retrieve and secure the body and carry her out to a waiting ambulance.

Then the park service handed Clayton Butler a notice of violation for BASE jumping in the park—which came with the possibility of a $5,000 fine and six months in jail. Two weeks later, federal prosecutors thought better of this and dismissed the charge. "To be sure, BASE jumping in Zion National Park is unlawful, and this tragic BASE jumping accident underscores some of the reasoning behind the regulations which prohibit such conduct in Zion National Park," said Melodyie Rydatch, spokeswoman for US attorney David Barlow. "Nevertheless, the interests of justice do not warrant prosecution of Mr. Butler."

"BASE jumping is so dangerous, even for those that are experienced, like Amber Bellows," acting park superintendent Jim Milestone told the *St. George News*. "That is one of the reasons it is not allowed in the park."

The danger is an issue, but it's not the main reason that the national parks do not permit BASE jumping and wingsuit jumping, a form of the sport that involves wearing a suit with fabric between the legs and under the arms to allow the jumper to soar like a flying squirrel. Since 1965 the Code of Federal Regulations has contained a section that bans parachuting from an aircraft, structure, or natural feature into a national park. The original spirit of the law was meant to prevent aerial delivery of cargo or people into the parks, but the National Park Service prohibits BASE jumping under this statute.

BASE jumpers say that this law forces them to jump at dusk and in other low-light situations to avoid detection by rangers, increasing the danger by obscuring their view of obstacles they may encounter between the jumper and the ground. "As the sun sets, shadows move over the land very rapidly," said BASE jumper Rick Harrison to a reporter from *High Country News* in July 2015. "It can really play tricks on you." He also said that those who jump in national parks often use old gear instead of their best equipment, because they fear that their gear will be confiscated if they are caught.

This is not what happened to Amber Bellows, but it may have played a role nearly five weeks later in the death of Sean Leary, a man with a solid reputation as "one of the most talented Yosemite climbers of his generation," a tribute in *Climbing* magazine tells us. Leary had scaled the 2,900-foot El Capitan in Yosemite National Park at least fifty times, including a record-setting scramble he completed in an astonishing two and a half hours—a route that takes mere mortals two to three days to complete. His BASE jumping included use of a wingsuit in remote spots all over the world, most notably in Patagonia, where he leaped from a 7,917-foot peak called El Mocho to scatter the ashes of Roberta Nunes, a friend who had died in an auto accident. Leary opened up "exits," a term for jumping-off points, in places as far away as Antarctica and above the Arctic Circle.

He arrived at Zion on March 13, 2014, with plans to jump in the West Temple area of the park that day and then meet up with a group of rock climbers the day after. When he did not arrive back home in California as scheduled on March 23, his family got in touch with the park. Park officials determined that Leary had not joined the climbers as scheduled on March 14.

As soon as word went out that Leary had gone missing in the park, fellow climbers, jumpers, and friends began to arrive at Zion to assist in the search.

"Hours later, Leary's body, rigged up in his BASE jumping gear, was found 300 feet beneath a high ridge in the park's West Temple area," the *Los Angeles Times* reported, adding, "He was 38 and about to become a father." The body was found in an aerial search using Grand Canyon's helicopter, in an area known as the Three Marys.

"Several of his experienced climbing friends were on standby to help move Leary to the top of the peak in case the helicopter had trouble reaching him," the park's news release said. "They also helped SAR rangers manage lines set up to reach Leary."

Recovery had to be postponed for several days because of harsh winds, but the team finally executed its plan to short-haul two rangers to a ledge above the body. They climbed down to Leary, rigged his remains for a long-line haul under the helicopter, and removed him from the remote area.

A lifelong climber who grew up in El Portal, California, virtually in the shadow of the High Sierra Mountains, Leary began BASE jumping in 2006 after Nunes's death, in part to ease the pain of loss. "I needed something that would take me to a different spot," he said in an interview. Later, he told filmmaker Chad Copeland, as quoted by the *Times*, "You're floating, you're floating—it's just magic when the wingsuit pops open and inflates and you start to take off."

The park service acknowledges this thrill, but it also remains firm in its prohibition of BASE jumping. "There are places within the United States that one can BASE jump, but not in Zion," acting park superintendent Jim Milestone said in the park's news release about the recovery mission. "There are many reasons for this, from resource protection, to visitor and employee safety, to Wilderness mandates. BASE jumping is not congruent with the founding purpose of this park."

Before we close this chapter, there's more to the story of Amber Bellows and Clayton Butler. On January 15, 2015, less than a year after Bellows fell to her death in Zion, Butler died while paragliding in Oahu, Hawaii. He fell from Kaena Point, on the westernmost tip of the island. Butler was thirty years old.

CHAPTER 6

Sudden Darkness:
The Zion–Mt. Carmel Tunnel

THE *ARIZONA REPUBLIC* WAXED ELOQUENT ON JULY 6, 1930, two days after the formal dedication of an engineering marvel in the heart of Zion National Park: "No highway completed in the west in a number of years has opened up the scenic beauty to motorists that a trip through the Mt. Carmel tunnel and the connecting roads affords . . . The new road, beginning near the park ranger station at the entrance, is only 26 miles long, but it is declared to be the most scenic in all America." In particular, the writer admired the road's new tunnels: "It incorporates two tunnels, one 5,600 feet long and the other more than 400 feet in length. These tunnels are cut through the crimson rock that forms the mountains, and some six galleries have been opened for ventilation and to afford motorists opportunities to view the wonderful panoramas that unfold before them as their cars emerge from the darkness."

Three years in the making at a cost of nearly $3 million (a value of more than $41 million in 2017 dollars), the new scenic highway and the Zion–Mt. Carmel Tunnel created a direct route from Zion to Bryce Canyon National Park to the northeast, and to Grand Canyon National Park to the south in Arizona, cutting the travel time to Bryce Canyon in half and shortening the time to Grand Canyon by a third. The National Park Service, the State of Utah, and the Bureau of Public Roads all had a hand in the project, but the vision for it came from National Park Service director Stephen Mather, who envisioned a "Grand Loop" highway that would become a "center of American tourism." The road through Zion was a small section of Mather's larger concept, but it formed a critical link that made a motor tour of Utah's parks accessible and affordable for millions of tourists. It also opened an area of the park that only intrepid tourists on foot or horseback had any chance of seeing before: Pine Creek Canyon and the eastern plateau, a world of vertical Navajo sandstone formations and planes of variegated slickrock.

The tunnel itself presented one of the road's greatest challenges. At the time of its construction, the 1.1-mile tunnel was the longest underground passageway in the national park system, and the engineering involved in its planning and construction pioneered new techniques that made this tunnel a manmade marvel in an extraordinary natural wilderness. The Nevada Contracting Company took on the challenge of actually building the tunnel under the supervision of expert crew bosses from across the country. They began by blasting gallery openings into the soft sandstone, creating a literal window in the side of the rock face through which they could reach the wall's interior. Carefully carving out the tunnel and removing rock, dirt, and sand through these windows, the crews burrowed out a narrow shaft from one end of the tunnel to the other, and then began the long, meticulous process of widening and shaping the tunnel from the inside.

It was during this construction that accidents began to happen—including two incidents that took the lives of diligent workmen.

The only way to remove large areas of rock during the construction was with the use of dynamite, blasting huge boulders into smaller rocks that could be hauled away or allowed to drop below the roadway and into the canyon. Blasting, however, came with its own side effects: The reverberations and destruction of sandstone layers caused rockslides, with rocks and dirt rolling uncontrolled through the work area.

Just such a rockfall caught Allan T. McClain, a thirty-five-year-old worker from Cleveland, Ohio, on January 19, 1928. McClain was operating a steam shovel when a rock fell from a ledge above him, crushing him against the machine. "The accident occurred at 3 o'clock on Wednesday afternoon, and he was immediately taken to a doctor," the *Iron County Record* reported, "but his lungs were so badly crushed, and possibly other internal injuries, that he died at three o'clock the next morning."

Only one other person had the misfortune to perish during the massive construction project. Johnny Morrison, a crew boss, died in the pilot tunnel—the small shaft the crews drilled to set the course of the tunnel before "ring drilling" the entire breadth, height, and width of the final opening. Knowing that workers would need adequate ventilation to labor in this narrow space, the project bosses planned five windows, or galleries, along the length of the tunnel as work progressed. On the night of July 1, 1928, crews blasted through the rock to open a connection between the third and fourth galleries, creating a particularly dramatic amount of sand and toxic dynamite fumes. Morrison was overcome and did not survive.

Given the size, scope, and topography of the project, we can consider it remarkable that these were the only two deaths among the workers.

Once the tunnel opened, twenty-eight years passed before Zion saw its first fatality from traffic—and this first death falls under the heading of "freak accident." Mrs. Milo D. Long of San Jose, California, stood posing for a photo in one of the tunnel's scenic gallery windows when she inexplicably lost her balance. She tumbled over the three-foot-high rock wall at the base of the window and plunged downward through the window and into the canyon below while her husband, who was holding the camera, watched in disbelief. "County Sheriff Roy A. Renouf said no inquest would be held in the mishap," the *Deseret News* reported two days later.

THE SOUTH WALL

With the advent of the interstate highway system in the 1950s and America's newfound love of the road trip in the 1960s and 1970s, traffic through Zion and many other national parks increased significantly. Zion officials began to realize that the curved nature of the Zion–Mt. Carmel Tunnel along its 1.1-mile length had not been planned to accommodate the volume of large, fast cars and trucks moving through it on a daily basis.

The tunnel's darkness and curves took their first victim in 1972, when twenty-one-year-old motorcycle rider Steven Michael Rose of Santa Rosa, California, lost control of his cycle as he entered the tunnel. "Officers say he drove the cycle into the tunnel wall," United Press International reported on June 7. "The tunnel leads through a mountainside to the lower level of the park and is not lighted."

In 1974 a second motorcycle death occurred, this time when three riders crashed into the tunnel's south wall at a point where it curves to the right. Harvey Frank Hoff, twenty-nine, of Phoenix died in the crash, and two other Phoenix visitors were injured: Brad Martin, twenty-one, and Roy W. Bieghler, thirty-two. The accident took place over Memorial Day weekend, a particularly crowded time in all of the western national parks. In all, eight riders were on a motorcycle trip together through the Utah parks when the crash occurred, according to a lawsuit filed in 1980 by the injured Bieghler and Hoff's widow, Joanne. Ms. Hoff and Bieghler sought damages for what they deemed to be negligence on the park's part, alleging "negligence in the design, construction, operation and maintenance of the tunnel." The court ruled in favor of the United States, preventing the case from going to trial, but the Court of Appeals for the Ninth Circuit in Phoenix overturned the lower court's decision. The appellate court based this on the testimony of an accident reconstruction expert, whose examination of the tunnel led him to conclude that the crash was due to negligence on the part of the Department of the Interior, because the inside of the tunnel did not have adequate lighting. This landmark decision, one quoted in dozens of cases that followed, allowed the plaintiffs to go to trial.

The case came to trial in 1982. Bieghler and Hoff's attorney, John H. Westover, claimed that the tunnel was a "deathtrap," according to United Press International's coverage of the trial, published in the *Arizona Republic*. "This tunnel is extremely dark and dangerous," he said in court. "It is a trap that catches victims, and it is one that caught Mr. Bieghler and Mr. Hoff." The $4.5 million lawsuit was filed in the US district court in Phoenix. Westover added that the tunnel was lighted by holes that let in sunlight, and that a flash of sunlight coming through the hole at the curve "temporarily blinded the motorcyclists."

Representing the federal government, US attorney Paul A. Katz wrote in a pretrial brief, "The United States will demonstrate that this tunnel has a remarkable safety record over its 50-year life." He noted that the three cyclists had taken their engines out of gear and were coasting on the downhill slope at speeds much faster than are recommended for the tunnel.

So how did this case turn out? I did my best to find the answer. When the Lexis/Nexis database contained no record of the trial, I contacted the US District Court in Phoenix, who told me that a case this old is no longer in an accessible file. The record of it, should it still exist on paper, is locked away in a warehouse that probably resembles the one at the end of the film *Raiders of the Lost Ark*. I could pay an exorbitant fee to have someone dig it out, but there is a good possibility it's not there at all. I even tried to contact

Bieghler through his Facebook page, but to date he has not responded. Sadly, the *Arizona Republic* did not report on the outcome either. We can only conclude that the case was settled quietly, perhaps even out of court, and that the end result did not warrant a great deal of fanfare.

In 1986, James F. Cooke of Colorado City, Arizona, rode his bicycle into the Zion–Mt. Carmel Tunnel behind three friends, Helaman, Heber, and Guy Barlow, at about 3:45 p.m. on a sunny April 11. Seconds later, he crossed into the oncoming traffic lane and ran into the concrete south wall. A physician and registered nurse treated him at the scene of the accident, and park ranger emergency medical technicians summoned an ambulance to take him to the Dixie Regional Medical Center in St. George. Later, the nature of his injuries made doctors decide to airlift him to a hospital in Las Vegas. He died there of his injuries two days later.

By this time accidents in the tunnel had become a common occurrence, although only the ones described above resulted in fatalities. Most of the accidents involved large vehicles like trailers, motor homes, and tour buses, methods of transportation that were not part of the American experience back in the 1920s when designers first imagined the passageway through Zion's rock walls.

In early 1989 the Federal Highway Administration conducted a study that determined that large modern conveyances like trailers and trucks could not get around the tunnel's curves without crossing the center line. This put all oncoming traffic at risk, causing other vehicles to swerve into the tunnel walls or to collide head-on with these big rigs. A complete overhaul of the tunnel was neither practical nor affordable, so as the park's spring 1989 season began, the National Park Service put new rules in place to control traffic and ensure the safety of motorists. These rules are still in effect.

Today the park posts rangers at either end of the tunnel, so that they can convert traffic to one-way when larger vehicles have to pass through. Truckers and drivers of large recreational vehicles (eleven feet, four inches tall or taller, and seven feet, 10 inches wide or wider) pay a fifteen-dollar tunnel permit fee for this service when they enter the park—and nearly thirty thousand drivers of oversized vehicles now pay this fee each year, making this a solution that funds itself. As rangers are stationed at the tunnel only during daylight hours (you can find the schedule at www.nps.gov/zion/planyourvisit/the-zion-mount-carmel-tunnel.htm), drivers of large vehicles need to plan their trip through the tunnel when this one-way service is available.

In addition, the park prohibits the largest vehicles from using the tunnel at all: If your trailer, RV, or truck is more than thirteen feet, one inch tall, weighs more than fifty thousand pounds, or is more than forty feet long, you cannot drive it through the Zion–Mt. Carmel tunnel. Finally, pedestrians and bicycles are not allowed in the tunnel at all, and vehicles are not permitted to stop in the tunnel for photos (or for any other reason other than tied-up traffic).

Only three deaths have been reported in the tunnel since the stepped-up safety regulations went into effect, and all of these involved motorcycles. On July 16, 1994, twenty-nine-year-old Marco Dyer entered the tunnel on his way west, lost control of his vehicle, and slammed into the tunnel's south wall. When park EMTs arrived minutes later, Dyer already had no pulse and had stopped breathing, and his pupils were fixed and dilated. He did not respond to aggressive attempts to resuscitate him. Dixie Regional Medical Center directed the emergency team to stop attempting to resuscitate the victim.

A nearly identical accident took place almost ten years later, on March 28, 2004, when two motorcyclists died in the tunnel. Colin Robert Morrow of St. George and Aaron J. Padilla of Salt Lake City, both twenty-one years old, crashed into the wall of the tunnel at about 5:45 p.m. They were about eight hundred feet inside the tunnel when they reached the first curve and veered into oncoming traffic, hitting the wall a second later. State trooper Kevin Davis, interviewed by the Associated Press, said that the two men were traveling at "excessive speed" as they entered the tunnel, where the speed limit is twenty-five miles per hour. He also noted that the men were wearing helmets, though this did not save their lives in this case.

These were the last fatalities in the Zion–Mt. Carmel Tunnel as of this writing. It's worth noting that in 2014, a group of eight bicyclists made an illegal attempt to cycle through the tunnel on a crowded Friday afternoon, refusing the shuttle service arranged for them by the park. While four other cyclists in the group rode the shuttle, the eight biked off into the tunnel, apparently expecting to find that the shuttle was nothing more than an attempt to curtail their fun.

Instead, two of the cyclists ran into a tunnel wall and crashed.

"As soon as we rounded the corner, it was like pitch black," one of the cyclists told officials later, as reported in a Fox 13 news article. "That's when it happened . . . he was just lying there."

One of the injured cyclists was a fifty-one-year-old man from West Jordan, who was rushed by ambulance to a hospital. The other declined medical care.

"They were in a bad spot, and only two of the bikers had little flashers," the cyclist who made a statement went on. "I thought, 'Someone else is going to get killed.'" He went back to the eastern end of the tunnel to alert rangers to stop traffic and get help. "That was my first thought cause I didn't want anybody else to get hurt. It was really stupid what we'd done . . . I think we all learned our lesson and we now have to pay the price."

The eight rogue bicyclists received violation notices from the park rangers.

CHAPTER 7

Due Process: Deaths by
Suspicious Circumstances

James and Patricia Bottarini arrived in Zion
National Park in May 1997, on what James told family
members he planned as a "second honeymoon" for the couple. Married nearly a decade and living in Medford, New
Jersey, the two had recently appeared tense to their friends
and neighbors, and Patty's sister, Carolyn Howard-Jones,
suspected that they had run into some bumps in the road
in their marriage. No one knew anything for certain, however, and when the Bottarinis headed out to Las Vegas on
May 7 for a vacation involving some wilderness exploration
in Zion, none of them suspected that anything untoward
would happen to Patty.

On May 9, 1997, the Bottarinis got up, had breakfast,
and started up the four-mile Observation Point trail. "The
hike from the Weeping Rock Trailhead to Observation
Point is a Zion classic, and the viewpoint at the end of the
trail is an iconic image of Zion National Park," notes Joe
Braun on his trail information website, Joe's Guide to Zion

National Park. The eight-mile round-trip hike "involves a lot of unrelenting uphill on a hard paved trail that was blasted out of the canyon walls . . . While this hike isn't as exposed or fear-inducing as Angels Landing, with an elevation gain of over 2,100 feet, Observation Point is a more strenuous workout."

They made it about three-quarters of the way to the top of the peak when they stopped for a snack and a few minutes of admiring the already spectacular view. At that point they decided they'd had enough of climbing and were too tired to reach the top, so they turned around and started back.

What exactly happened next became the center of speculation and an investigation that continued for more than half a decade.

James would tell authorities and a courtroom that he got ahead of Patricia on the narrow trail, walking fifteen feet or more in front of her. "Something had alerted me to turn around," he said in an account of the event five years later, "whether she had called me or whatever." He said he turned to see Patty lying facedown on the sloped ledge. She was scrambling to get back up when she lost her footing. James said that in the space of about two seconds, he saw her slip away over the edge and disappear. "She was sliding down," he said. "There was nowhere for her to stop."

At that moment Donald and Glenda Cox of Amarillo, Texas, were somewhat lower on the series of switchbacks leading up the trail. They had already hiked to the top and were on the descent when they paused to rest, and they heard "scuffling" sounds coming from about a mile above them. They looked up to see rocks falling off the cliff—and then, to their astonishment, they saw Patricia Bottarini fall over the edge. She was "cartwheeling like a cheerleader," Donald Cox said. Patricia's fall happened just a second or two after the sounds he and his wife had heard above them.

Glenda Cox grabbed her binoculars and tried to find where Patricia had landed, and the two of them waited to hear cries from above or some evidence that the falling woman had been with a companion on the trail. "We were waiting for someone to yell," Donald said. "Somebody had just fallen off a cliff, and we anticipated that somebody would do something, would say something."

After several minutes it became clear to the Coxes that it was up to them to report the incident. They rushed to the trailhead, got in their car, and drove to the park's visitor center to alert rangers to what they had seen.

Meanwhile, a group of six hikers from Phoenix—Robert Falk, Mike Fulton, their female hiking partners, and two others—stopped suddenly on the Observation Point trail when they encountered a confused and visibly shaken James Bottarini coming toward them. James told them that his wife had fallen and he could not find her. Fulton offered him a topographical map, but in a moment the group realized that this was not a case of someone wandering away. James didn't express any "sense of panic or urgency," Fulton said later. The rattled husband seemed unable to help them make plans to search for Patty, and he didn't say much—but his voice quivered and his hands trembled, sure signs that something was terribly wrong.

Falk would tell authorities later that James did not call out Patty's name as they searched for her, leaving that task to him. He seemed distracted and disoriented, and did not help significantly with the search. When Falk hoisted himself up on a ledge covered with loose soil, he came upon something he would never forget: Patricia's body, broken and bloody where she had fallen some five hundred feet from the trail above.

"It was not something anyone should see," he testified in court more than five years later. "It was instantly a situation where I knew we wouldn't be able to help her." He immediately did his best to keep James from seeing his wife's condition. "I turned to [Jim] and said something to the effect of, 'Jim, it's not good, don't come up here.'"

Falk knelt down to check to see if Patty was breathing and heard James's footsteps behind him. He knew that James was looking at the body, but the man showed little emotion at seeing his wife this way. "He did, however, pick up a rock and throw it at a pack of vultures circling overhead," the *Deseret News* noted in its coverage of the incident. When Falk determined that someone should head back to find authorities and report the accident, James told him that he "needed to stay" with his wife. Falk dispatched his girlfriend and others to run back to the trailhead three miles away and go find help; when he returned to James, he noted that James had replaced Patty's shorts, which had come off in the fall.

As they sat together and waited for rangers to arrive, Falk learned that the Bottarinis had two young sons, one three years old and one nine months old. James put his head in his hands and cried for a time, and he expressed concern about what it would take to remove Patty's body from the ledge.

National Park Service ranger Brett McGinn was the first to arrive on the scene, finding Falk and James Bottarini waiting for him. James seemed "emotionally separated" from what was going on, McGinn said. "I had questions as to James Bottarini's attitude and demeanor. He seemed to be detached and disinterested from what was going on." James barely spoke as the rescue workers recovered Patricia's body, though he broke down and cried when he mentioned his children and how difficult this would be for them.

Special agent Pat Buccello described a similar observation of Bottarini as she questioned him at the scene. At first she mistook Falk for the husband, because he seemed more worried and upset than Bottarini. Then she and the park rangers on the scene began to realize that something very strange had taken place here. "We all kind of looked at each other and said, 'Nobody falls off Observation Point Trail,'" she said. She went so far as to check park records later that day, and found she was right: There had been no accidents on this trail in the past thirty years, and no fatalities in the sixty years the trail had been open.

The following day, as detectives began to piece together what happened, they realized that they might have a case against James Bottarini.

They interviewed Carolyn Howard-Jones and asked her if she thought her sister was the victim of an accident. "I could not say yes, and I could not say no," she told them. She said that when James told her of Patty's death, "It was very matter of fact. It was as if he was reading something off of a piece of paper." He told her two different stories: First, he said the couple was hiking the Angels Landing trail when he suddenly heard Patricia call out, and turned to see that she had fallen. Later, James told her that they were hiking the Observation Point trail and when he heard her slip, he turned around to see her sliding off the edge and "screaming" for him to do something.

Soon investigators discovered that Patricia had made James the beneficiary of a $250,000 life insurance policy and more than $1 million in her share of her family's California real estate business. On the day Patricia died and again a few weeks later, James told Buccello the name of the life insurance company and the amount of Patricia's coverage, but in a taped phone conversation with Buccello in July, he denied that he knew any of this information and said he hadn't even known Patricia had life insurance.

Five days after Patricia's fall, investigators discovered an unusual blood spot about eight feet down the cliff. No impact marks preceded that particular spot, although Washington County undersheriff Peter Kuhlmann found drag marks at five feet and twenty-five feet from the blood spot. He found these to be "consistent with what I would expect to see in a fall," he said. The one blood spot with no drag marks, however, suggested that Patricia may not have slid off the edge and tumbled down the slope; she might have sailed through the air before hitting the ground, as if she had been pushed.

Howard-Jones began to take a stand against James, refusing to allow him to stay at her Oceanside, California, home the week after Patty's death when he arrived there for her memorial service. Six months later, she refused to sign a letter saying that Patty's death was accidental. Patty's relatives challenged her will, filing a lawsuit to prevent any of the family trust from being disbursed to James, but their case was dismissed in October 2000.

With evidence pointing to the possibility of foul play, the federal government charged Bottarini with interstate domestic violence, making false statements to a federal officer, and four counts of mail fraud for attempting to collect on the insurance policy. If he was found guilty of the domestic violence charge, he faced the possibility of a lifetime prison sentence. The federal government did not have the authority to charge Bottarini with murder—that was up to the Washington County Sheriff's Office, and Washington County attorney Eric Ludlow told the *Deseret News* that he was "monitoring" the case, and would wait for the results before deciding whether to charge Bottarini in his wife's death.

When at last the case went to trial in federal court in November 2002—five years after Patricia's death—jury members were chosen based on their ability to walk the trail to Observation Point and see firsthand where Patricia had fallen. They made the five-hour bus trip from Salt Lake City, where the trial took place, to stand at the spot where Patricia had reached the end of her life and draw their own conclusions about how she had died.

The prosecution described James as "a systematic gambler who bet he could get away with murder." It portrayed him as a schemer who began his plot to kill his wife eight months before she died, when the couple took out life insurance policies and she prepared a will that favored James. The man was a controlling husband, the prosecution continued, with a risky investment business that was on the rocks. US attorney Richard Lambert also noted that Patricia was an excellent athlete, but that she had "a terrible fear of heights."

The defense dismissed all of these accusations, especially the ones that showcased Bottarini's demeanor on the day his wife died. James had behaved like a man in shock, said defense attorney Ronald Yengich. "If he had planned this, he would have been bawling all over the place," he said, underscoring that James's reaction to Patricia's death was inconsistent with someone who planned to kill his wife.

The prosecution presented evidence of James's penchant for gambling, including the frequency of his trips to Las Vegas while he lived in California—fifty-three visits between 1990 and 1994—and his accumulated losses of more than $73,000 between January 1995 and April 1997. Friends and family, however, testified that the Bottarinis both came from affluent families and did not have debt issues or a flamboyant lifestyle.

For three weeks forensic experts gave contradictory testimony about whether Patricia would have or could have stumbled and fallen over the edge of the switchback, and how she might have tumbled down the steep rock face. A professor of exercise science insisted that if Patricia had slipped or tripped, she would have fallen forward instead of sideways. A forensic engineer said that a wide range of issues, from vertigo to physical exhaustion, could have swayed Patricia as much as forty-five degrees in any direction. The prosecution pushed for claims that Patricia's fear of heights would have made her avoid the edge, while the defense showed photos of Patricia rappelling down a rock face, implying that the prosecution exaggerated Patricia's phobia—if she had one at all.

Blood spatter experts disagreed on whether the blood-stains found at the scene could tell them whether Patricia had slipped and fallen down the canyon wall, or whether she had been pushed and had fallen through the air. One said that she was already bleeding before she fell, and that four bloodstains in an elliptical pattern showed that she was "vaulted out" over the edge of the cliff. Another said that the patterns were consistent with a tumble after slipping and falling, and abrasions on Patricia's hands were consistent with testimony that she simply slipped and fell. This dis-agreement became a central focus of the case for the defense: "How she fell I don't know, and [prosecutors] don't know," Yengich said in his closing statement. "There's reasonable doubt there. This is about a tragedy that occurred in a world that does not exist in blacks and whites. There are shades of gray, and accidents do happen."

James Bottarini concurred, testifying on his own behalf on the last two days of the trial. "I did not kill my wife," he said, his eyes filled with tears. "There's no possible way that I would want my wife dead."

On Tuesday, November 26, 2002, after ten hours of deliberation, jurors in the case handed down their verdict: They acquitted James Bottarini of all the charges against him. One of the jurors told the media that the acquittals were the "result of a misunderstanding rather than an over-whelming sense of Bottarini's innocence," reporter Angie Welling wrote in the *Deseret News* on December 4. The juror told Welling that the jury misread the lengthy instructions they were given by the judge and believed that "their inability to come to a unanimous verdict of guilt had to result in a default acquittal." Ten of the twelve jurors believed that Bottarini killed his wife, the juror said, but still found him not guilty because they believed they were not permitted to let the trial end with a hung jury.

The juror's statement to the media opened the door to additional speculation and ways to find a court that would rule that Bottarini was guilty. Civil lawsuits from Patricia's family, the insurance company, and the guardian appointed to see to the children's financial affairs continued to follow Bottarini for years following his acquittal, both to prevent him from receiving any benefits from his wife's death and to attempt to find him responsible for the death in the less stringent forum of a civil court, where a majority of jurors—rather than a unanimous jury—could find him guilty.

I contacted the Superior Court of California and obtained a copy of the February 10, 2005 decision in the case brought by TOBO Investment Partnership, the real estate company owned by Patricia's family, against James Bottarini, and the cross-complaint Bottarini filed against TOBO Investments. The cross-complaint also named David H. Dougan III, the guardian ad litem appointed by the court to represent the Bottarinis' two sons.

In the settlement agreement, James Bottarini dropped his countersuit against Dougan, and Dougan waived the boys' rights to the property owned by Patricia's family. Most significant, however, is item 4 in the terms of the agreement: "Each party hereto agrees that the promises, covenants, and releases contained herein are not, and are not to be deemed or constructed as, an admission of any misconduct or fault of any kind whatsoever; but are to be constructed strictly as a compromise and settlement of all disputes between the parties for the purpose of avoiding further controversy, litigation, and expense."

So the civil court did not retry Bottarini for his wife's death, and he and his sons received no proceeds from his wife's family's business interests. And that, apparently, was the end of that.

A Tent in the River

When twenty-three-year-old Arizona State University senior John Goebel and his friend Sarah Toler embarked on a spring break camping trip to Zion National Park in 2004, they probably planned a quiet week of hiking and exploring throughout the magnificent park.

On the evening of March 15, however, two campers from Alaska heard the friends arguing in their campsite near the Virgin River, just outside the park. They kept an eye on the situation, and around midnight they determined that Goebel was not entirely in control of himself. They "helped Goebel into his tent," they would later explain to authorities, and bedded down in their own tent for the night.

"When they woke up, his tent was gone," Washington County sheriff's chief deputy Rob Tersigni told the media days later. "They figured he had gone hiking or something."

Thirty-six hours passed, but Goebel did not return. Toler finally reported to authorities that he was missing at 10:30 a.m. on Wednesday, March 17. She apparently left the park soon after, perhaps believing that her friend had deserted her in the park.

The next morning, police found a zipped-up tent lying in the Virgin River, pressed up against a large rock. Goebel's body was inside.

Toler turned up in a bus station in Las Vegas, where police took her into custody and questioned her. She told them that Goebel had been drinking heavily on the evening of March 15, and tried to pressure her into having "more of a relationship." She assured him she was not interested in this. She enlisted the two men from Alaska to help her get Goebel into his sleeping bag, and went to sleep in her own. None of them saw Goebel again.

A medical examination determined that Goebel had water in his lungs, but the medical examiner did not say conclusively that he had drowned. Authorities believe he died sometime on Tuesday, March 16.

Toler was released and was "not considered a suspect," according to Tersigni.

Goebel did not appear to have any significant trauma on his body, so the medical examiner proceeded with toxicology tests. While the Utah medical examiner does not share results with the media, the sheriff's office in Springdale did inform me that based on the medical examiner's report, the death was ruled an accident.

CHAPTER 8

On the Road: Vehicular Deaths

ON A SUNNY SUNDAY AFTERNOON IN AUGUST 1937, TWENTY-two-year-old Clair L. Hirschi of Rockville, Utah, chose to enjoy the day with a motorcycle ride through Zion National Park.

When he reached the turn onto the Virgin River bridge at the intersection of the canyon highway and the Zion–Mt. Carmel Tunnel road, he failed to negotiate the turn. Hirschi and his motorcycle plunged over the embankment and fell into the canyon at machine speed.

People who saw the accident acted quickly to summon help, but when emergency personnel arrived and transported Hirschi to Zion Lodge, the nurse in charge there had no choice but to pronounce him dead. The staff summoned Dr. E. Clark McIntyre from Hurricane to make the final diagnosis: Hirschi had died on impact of a broken neck, apparently because he was not experienced in riding and handling this particular vehicle.

The story of a young man dying needlessly on a summer day would be sad enough, but on closer examination, the Hirschi story dives to unusual lows. Clair Hirschi left behind a young wife and a two-month-old baby. Ten days earlier, his father, Heber, had attended a baseball game at a tournament in nearby Hurricane, and found himself in the path of a fly ball that struck the side of his head, leaving him with a severe injury. And a day after that, Clair's younger brother Arden "was badly injured by a runaway team at Grafton," the *Washington County News* reported. Another media source said that Arden died of his injuries as well.

Fortunately, young Mrs. Hirschi's parents arrived from California for the funeral (along with many other out-of-town relatives, friends, and even staff members of the local paper, at what was reported to be a very well-attended event), and we can hope that they were ready to look after the young bride and her baby thereafter.

While motor vehicle accidents are not uncommon in Zion—motorists staring at magnificent views instead of at the road find themselves in fender benders and minor mishaps along the park's scenic drives—I could find only three that actually resulted in a death in the park. This does not include the ones that took place in the Zion–Mt. Carmel Tunnel (detailed in chapter 6), although these still add only five deaths to the list.

Those who met their end in a motor vehicle include assistant chief ranger Fred E. Bergemeyer, a thirty-nine-year-old firefighter on his way to do his valuable and courageous job in the park on August 23, 1952. While rushing to "a fire reportedly burning high on the east rim of the canyon" at about 4:30 p.m. on a rugged park trail used only for firefighting, the weapons carrier he was driving hit a patch of mud. He lost control and the rig flipped over and rolled, killing Bergemeyer instantly.

Through a miraculous stroke of good fortune, park ranger Joseph Romberg, who was also in the vehicle, was not injured in the accident. He ran to an emergency telephone and called park headquarters for assistance, but nothing could be done for the assistant ranger. Bergemeyer grew up in Nora Springs, Iowa, graduated from Iowa State College at Ames, and had been a forest ranger ever since. He left behind his wife, Diane, and their two sons: Jerry, who was seven, and five-year-old Michael.

MYSTERY ROLLOVERS

Not every accident has a clear cause, and investigations do not always reveal answers. This was the case on July 23, 1967, when a family from Columbus, Ohio, suddenly veered off Utah Route 15 two miles inside Zion National Park and plummeted seventy feet to the bottom of a ravine.

In the front seat, Jean Helen Newman, who was thirty-seven years old, died at the scene of the accident. Her husband, John William Newman, was driving the vehicle and died two hours later in a hospital in Kanab. Their twelve-year-old son, John, survived the crash with only minor injuries, but United Press International reported that his younger brother Thomas, who was ten, was in critical condition the following day.

The media tells us no more about this family, and any record of a continuing investigation has long been lost.

An accident of a similar kind in 2013, however, made national news as the first of its kind in American history. On

July 26 the Model T Ford Club International held its annual driving tour in Zion National Park, and saw its first-ever accident with a fatality.

A 1915 Ford Model T, driven by a nineteen-year-old from Minnesota, pulled to the side of Utah Route 9 at about 10:20 a.m. to allow faster traffic to pass it on its way into the park. When the driver tried to get the vehicle back onto the pavement, investigators said, he "didn't negotiate the small dirt slope properly, and the added weight and stress on the tires caused the wooden spokes on the right front wheel to collapse."

Then "the vehicle flipped," the Utah Highway Patrol reported to the Associated Press. Sergeant LaMar Heaton said to the *Deseret News*, "A modern car with the safety features . . . it wouldn't have had any problem getting back on the road."

The Model T did not have seat belts, but this may have been irrelevant, Model T experts interviewed by the AP said. "Restraints are of little use in the soft-top vehicle that typically travels at no more than 30 mph," according to the article. Added Andy Loso, vice president of the Minnesota T-Totalers club, "There's no rollover protection."

Four people were in the antique automobile, which had a soft top that was crushed in the accident. All four were ejected from the vehicle, and fifty-one-year-old Karen Johnson, president of the T-Totalers car club in Minnesota, was seriously injured. Paramedics worked for an hour to try to revive her at the scene, but she did not regain consciousness.

Johnson's husband, Tim, was in another antique car some distance ahead, trooper Jalaine Hawkes reported to the *Deseret News*. He came back to find her and learned the news of the accident, and he was at her side as she was air-lifted to the nearest hospital, where she passed away.

The other passengers included the Johnsons' son and twelve-year-old granddaughter, as well as the driver. They all suffered injuries but survived the incident.

Tour chairman Russ Furstnow said that the club members—many of whom were in attendance and driving the 170 Model T Fords in the tour—were "extremely upset about the whole thing." He said the club, which has members all over the world, is "a family," and there had never been an accident on one of its tours.

That summer, the club had driven along the Grand Canyon and on the seventeen-mile driving route in Bryce Canyon National Park. "The Model T is just a social medium," he said. "It brings people together that have a love for these old cars. We have these summer reunions and it's almost like an extended family."

Karen Johnson was "outgoing, caring, just a wonderful lady—a definite sparkplug," Furstnow told the *Minneapolis Star-Tribune*, which reaches the Johnsons' hometown of Owatonna, Minnesota.

Loso noted that the Johnsons worked together restoring cars, and that they did an excellent job maintaining their vehicles. "Karen was always in the garage working on things, getting dirty. She'd grab the other women and bring them in and try to teach them stuff."

WRECKAGE ON A RAINY NIGHT

In a Friday night rainstorm on the northeast boundary of Zion's northernmost unit, Kolob Canyon, the pilot of a single-engine Cessna 172RG reported that the plane was "taking on ice."

The message came through to the Los Angeles Flight Control Center at 7:56 p.m. on November 6, 1987, just before the plane disappeared from radar. The pilot, twenty-four-year-old Brad Woolsey, also radioed that clouds now obscured his vision. He abruptly descended from 10,500 feet to 8,500 feet, bringing the plane into direct line with the terrain on the canyon edge.

The plane had left Prescott, Arizona, for a flight to Rexburg, Idaho, with passengers Glen Campbell, who was twenty-three, and twenty-four-year-old Michelle Keller. Before takeoff the pilot was briefed about light to moderate rime icing in the clouds and precipitation, and he learned that the freezing level was forecast to be at about seven thousand to nine thousand feet in the Prescott area—and lower as the plane traveled north. Woolsey maintained regular contact with flight control, gathered additional weather information, and finally indicated that he would head to Cedar City rather than continue to Idaho that night.

"At 1962 MST, the pilot inquired about the distance to Cedar City and was told it was at his one o'clock position at 23 miles," the NTSB transcript reads (I've spelled out the abbreviations in this transcript). "He acknowledged and this was his last known transmission."

A search on Monday, November 9, used the "computer footprints" created by the Cessna's altitude and coding transponder and sent to the Flight Control Center in Los Angeles as it entered the park. A pilot from the Civil Air Patrol in Salt Lake City and an army helicopter from Dugway

Proving Ground, ninety miles southwest of Salt Lake City, followed these signals to the crash site in the canyon.

"We had a pilot flying these precise footprints as it entered the park," said Lieutenant Robert Smith of the Civil Air Patrol to the *Arizona Republic*. "Then he flew the plane wherever it would go after reaching that last point." The lower-flying helicopter assisted the pilot and ground crews—including search and rescue personnel on horseback and in all-terrain vehicles—in locating the wreckage. Working together, the Washington County search teams found the crashed plane at about 2:00 p.m., and reached it by 3:00 p.m. The pilot and the two passengers had died in the crash.

"It collided with trees on wooded terrain at an elevation of about 8050'," the NTSB transcript concluded. "No pre-impact mechanical problem was found."

A dark night, high terrain, adverse weather, a low cloud ceiling, and the trees were all factors in bringing this plane down on the edge of Zion's high country, according to the NTSB report.

CHAPTER 9

Unclassified:
Deaths by Unusual Causes

BACK BEFORE ZION BECAME A NATIONAL PARK, THE CAN-yon served as a cornucopia of natural resources for the handful of hardy souls who chose to settle there. It provided fresh water for growing food and hydrating livestock, stone for solid foundations of homes, and trees that could become lumber for building shelters, barns, and fences to allow settlers to establish homesteads in this gorgeous landscape. The new arrivals in the late 1890s and early 1900s chose this rugged place despite the potential hardships of drought, rock slides, intense summer heat, and difficulty in obtaining goods and materials that made living easier in America at the turn of the twentieth century. They wanted a different kind of life, and they were not afraid of the hard physical labor required to achieve it.

One of the tools the settlers created was the cable works, a mechanism to convey lumber from the vast yellow pine forest at the top of the canyon down to the burgeoning town below. David Flanigan, one of the residents, built a sawmill at the mountaintop, but he needed a way to bring his freshly hewn lumber down to the waiting families in Springdale and beyond. He came up with the idea for a cable transport system that used a pulley at the top to allow loads to travel smoothly downward at a controlled pace.

The first structure, according to the history book *Zion National Park* by Tiffany Taylor, "contained a 12-foot-high by 8.5-foot-wide cribbing of sawn, squared timbers—each measuring 10 inches in diameter. This cribbing was joined together by dowels and contained a pulley over which the cable wire ran. The pulley had two tracks for the wire, and a braking mechanism was located about 30 feet to the side of the structure."

A second cable draw works, built in 1901, added "a large platform for the cable operator [and] a smaller, manually operated pulley that was used to haul lumber to the platform, where it could be loaded in baskets and sent down the canyon." The cable works became a great success—so much so that by December 1906, Flanigan had conveyed two hundred thousand feet of sawn lumber from the top of what became known as Cable Mountain to the canyon floor. (Media coverage at the time consistently calls this distance three thousand feet; the park says this distance is actually two thousand feet.)

The system had one fairly dangerous flaw, however: It attracted lightning. As the highest thing on an already high point, it invited bolts to hit it in stormy weather—and storms often arrived with little or no warning in the days before Doppler radar and sophisticated forecasting.

On July 28, 1908, a group of young people from Springdale visited the cable works to see the mighty machines in action. Among them were Clarinda Langston, Thornton Hepworth Jr., and Lionel Stout, all of whom were about nine years old. Young Stout was the son of one of the lumbermen who worked at the top of the mountain, and Lionel was up there that day as well, working alongside his father.

As the three children stood and watched the lumber platform make its way down the canyon on strong metal wires, a bolt of lightning snaked out and hit the cable works. The two boys fell to the ground, and Clarinda found herself blinded by the electrical charge. "I did not know what was happening and I went blind and couldn't see," she was quoted later.

Someone spread a quilt under a tree and led Clarinda to it, urging her to sit or lie down and wait there in safety. When people rushed to help Lionel and Thornton, they found both young boys had been killed by the blast.

"Their bodies were taken down the mountain using the cable works," Taylor wrote—an act acknowledging just how rustic the Zion area was, with no road to bring the boys down to their families.

The tragedy did not stop progress. The cable works continued to operate until 1927, transporting lumber down from the sawmill at the top of the mountain.

Fire on Cable Mountain

Clarence Lemmon and Ether Winder were working at the top of Cable Mountain on Sunday, December 18, 1921, to bring back a load of lumber, an arduous task even with use of the cable system. The two young men—Winder was just shy of twenty-one years old—worked through the night to mill and load their lumber, and continued working through the day on Sunday in a soaking rain and, eventually, a wet snow that chilled them through to the bone. Winder had camped in a sheep wagon until that Sunday evening, when Lemmon invited him into his brother David's house—"a good substantial dwelling house that I lived in during the summer while operating the mill and was well furnished and contained a good store of supplies," David Lemmon wrote to the *Washington County News* on January 10, 1922, in a letter also signed by Enos E. Winder, Eliel Winder, and John A. Allred.

Knowing that he needed to dry his clothes and eager to sleep in a warm place instead of in a wagon surrounded by ten inches of new-fallen snow, Winder gratefully accepted the invitation. He carried his bedding out of the wagon and made himself a place on the floor of the main room of the house. Clarence Lemmon made them some supper (David was not there), and the young men built a strong fire, hung their clothes up to dry, and got some rest after their long, hard night and day.

Winder awoke with a start at about 10:30 p.m. to discover that the house was on fire. He yelled for Lemmon to wake up and run and bolted out of the shack himself. Lemmon woke up and realized that the fire had already burned through the partition between the two rooms and the flames had reached the foot of his bed. He got up and ran, rushing right over Winder's bed on his way out of the cabin and noting with relief that Winder was not in the bed. For a few precious seconds, he believed that both of them had escaped unharmed.

Suddenly he heard groaning from inside the house. Lemmon ran back into the burning building and discovered Winder lying across Lemmon's bed. Winder, not seeing his friend outside because of all the smoke billowing between them, had run back in to save Lemmon from the fire. Once inside, however, as he felt his way to the bedroom and pawed at the bed to find Lemmon, he was overcome by the smoke almost immediately and collapsed across the bed.

Clarence "caught Winder about the waist and pulled him off the bed," David Lemmon's letter continued, "however Winder being a large man, he was unable to lift him and by this time the fire had cut off all possible retreat by way of the door so he was obliged to make his retreat through the window." With smoke and flames threatening to consume him, Clarence finally had no choice but to abandon Winder's body and run for his life. Clarence told his brother that "he [knew] that Winder was dead when he pulled him from the bed."

Clarence ran for his horse and rode two miles in wind and snow, clad only in his union suit, to the nearest phone to call the people of Springdale. He reached John Winder, Ether's father, who told him to wait where he was for help to arrive and to keep warm until they could bring him some clothing.

John Winder rounded up a rescue party in minutes, bringing six people—his sons Elmer and Lyle; neighbors Hyrum Orin, Howard Ruesch, and Alvin Allred; and Clarence's brother, David—up the trail in Zion Canyon to the top of the mountain. When they arrived at about 2:45 a.m., only smoldering timber remained of the house. "Ether's body was found with the head resting under the springs of Clarence Lemmon's bed. It was badly charred, the head, lower part of the arms and part of the legs being entirely consumed by the fire," the *Washington County News* reported later that week.

Witnesses concluded that the fire "very likely was started from the stove pipe in the ceiling," the *County News* said. The men who wrote the impassioned letter to the *County News* ended their account with an admonishment: "There seems to be a tendency on the part of some to cast reflections upon young Lemmon for this disaster. You can see from the above that no blame can be attached to anyone."

A FINAL CABLE MOUNTAIN CASUALTY

Even after it fell into disuse in 1927, the cable line had one more act of destruction left in its system.

On April 11, 1930, Orderville school principal Albin Brooksby took a group of students on an outing in Zion Canyon, including a picnic and outdoor activities in the shadow of the old cable system. Long since dormant by that time, the cable stood only as a historical marker and most of it had been disassembled, but one piece remained in place: the iron clevis, a U-shaped fastener that was the central part of a pinning device. The large piece of iron appeared to be secured at the top of the cable.

As the students and their principal enjoyed their picnic under the former cable system, the ten-pound iron clevis suddenly came free and slid down three thousand feet of cable, gaining "terrific speed" on its way down the nearly vertical drop. It crashed into the group at the base at literally terminal velocity.

"The clevice [sic] struck Brooksby first, hitting him on the head and body and nearly cutting him in half," the *Washington County News* said the following week, "then went through the boys, breaking the arm and collar bone of Eugene Russell and cutting his face." The device also lacerated the skull of another boy, Lee Stevens, and several other boys received less serious cuts and bruises. Henry Carroll, an Orderville resident, took the two gravely injured boys to the Iron County hospital, where Russell remained overnight. Stevens was able to return home that evening.

A prominent citizen in the small Utah community, Brooksby was a member of the bishopric of his ward of the Church of Jesus Christ of Latter-day Saints, and served as a Scout leader. He left behind a wife and four children.

"Today, all that survives of the Draw Works system is the upper terminal," the park's website tells us. "The towers on the canyon floor and the cable were removed within a few years of the end of operation." The remaining structure was listed on the National Register of Historic Places in 1978, and the park completed a stabilization project in 2011 to preserve this landmark.

ONE CCC INJURY ENDS IN DEATH

From 1933 through 1942, the Civilian Conservation Corps came to Zion to complete public works projects that taught young men skills to make them employable for the rest of their lives. CCC workers in Zion built trails, campgrounds, and parking areas; constructed buildings still in use today; assisted in firefighting; and reduced the flooding of the Virgin River.

Most of their work required strong bodies that could handle hard labor like removing trees, digging trenches, and hefting building supplies; some men also learned to use explosives like dynamite as they blasted out rock walls to create open areas. Remarkably, only one of these men lost his life in such a pursuit—and he wasn't even handling the explosives.

Seventeen-year-old Ray Tanner walked into a blasting area near the Bridge Mountain CCC camp on December 28, 1937, just as the men there set off a charge. "His leg was nearly severed from his body by a large rock that flew more than three hundred feet to strike him as he was leaving a small building near the work project," the *Washington County News* said.

A resident of Salem, Utah, Tanner had arrived at the camp just two weeks before the accident occurred. Medics at the camp gave him first aid, and camp surgeons I. F. Clark and Von H. Robertson rushed him off to Fort Douglas hospital. There he went directly into emergency amputation surgery and survived the ordeal, but "surgical shock" and a severe infection set in soon after. His body gave up the fight on February 8, 1938, six weeks after the accident.

"On the day that notice of their fellow enrollee's death was received by the members of the camp, they did a memorial retreat formation in his honor," the newspaper reported. The men of the CCC stood at attention and dipped the United States flag as one of their number played "Taps" on a horn. They also sent a floral wreath to Tanner's parents, and five members of the corps attended his funeral in Salem.

"On January 31, the company made up a sum of $25.90 in donation to be mailed to enrollee Tanner," the *Washington County News* continued. "This was mailed in a cashier's check on the day of his death." We can probably assume this uncommon generosity—given that these men were only paid $30 per month, and sent $25 of this home to their families—eventually found its way to Tanner's family to help cover the cost of the funeral.

DEATH BY CHOICE

There are those who take their work with them on vacation, whether they visit a national park, make their way to a tropical island, or spend their time off with relatives and friends. Conversely, there are those whose work finds them wherever they go. Such was the case when a vacationing Los Angeles police detective came upon the decomposing body of a young woman on July 1, 1947, in the Emerald Pools area of Zion National Park.

If the discerning eye of an experienced detective had not happened upon the woman, she might never have been found at all, lying as she was off the trail in some brush.

The woman turned out to be Evelyn Frances Callahan, an identification made when Sheriff A. B. Prince of Washington County sent her fingerprints to the FBI laboratory in Washington, DC. The twenty-three-year-old woman was employed by Pacific Telegraph and Telephone Company in Seattle, Washington. On December 16, 1946, she had transferred within the company to Portland, Oregon—and on June 5, 1947, she had abruptly resigned her position, and had not been heard from since.

Sheriff's office investigators found two items near the body that helped them begin to piece together the young woman's story. First, they discovered shreds of a Zion Park tour ticket in the name of Mary McCafferty. The second item was a .32-caliber pistol. The county coroner quickly determined that Callahan had died of a gunshot wound to the head, a fact corroborated by the FBI's investigation of the scene. The federal bureau decided, however, that the position of the gun and the direction from which the bullet entered the body ruled out suicide. "A coroner's jury reached a verdict that the woman met her death by foul play," the *Deseret News* reported ten days later.

As to a slayer, however, there seemed to be no clues at all. Who was Mary McCafferty, and if she played a role in Callahan's death, why would she so carelessly leave her ticket and her weapon behind?

Working with the FBI, the sheriff began to form another theory. He discovered that a woman matching Callahan's description had arrived in Cedar City on June 13, 1947, and registered at the Leigh Hotel. Her registration, however, was in the name Mary McCafferty. The name appeared again on the tour bus passenger list, but bus company officials said "this name was not checked back onto the bus for the return trip," a *Salt Lake Telegram* story said. Evelyn Callahan's name was not on the tour bus's list.

Waitresses in the park's lodge said that they believed they had seen Callahan with a man, leading the sheriff and the FBI to initiate a search throughout the western states. As the sheriff interviewed family members, however, his position on the cause of Callahan's death began to change.

He spoke with Hugh M. Callahan, Evelyn's brother, who gave him a new piece of information: Evelyn knew she was "suffering from a serious ailment." Sheriff Prince told the *Telegram* that this illness was "an incurable disease." Hugh also identified the pistol as one that he knew his sister had at the family home in Oregon.

Evelyn's mother, Ann Theressa Callahan, related all of the same details when the sheriff interviewed her. These revelations must have drawn the investigation to a close, as there is no more mention of it in the media of that era.

While a number of national parks have fairly high numbers of suicides that take place within their borders, Zion has only two others in its records. One, the death of Dorothy Kaiser in 2003, remained an unsolved case (as described in chapter 3), but it appears that she took her own life on Angels Landing.

The other is the quiet but spectacular death of David Brigham in an apparent leap from Canyon Overlook. Rangers came across Brigham's vehicle at the overlook trailhead on the evening of February 25, 2009, and seeing no evidence that anyone was on the trail, they began looking for him. They discovered his body at about 8:00 a.m. on Thursday, February 26, at the base of the Great Arch. Brigham had fallen about four hundred feet to his death.

"A preliminary investigation of the fatality by the Washington County Sheriff's Office and the National Park

Service has indicated that the death was most likely a suicide," the park's news release said. As is appropriate for this very personal act, no further details were forthcoming.

LOST IN HOP VALLEY

Few hikers familiar with Zion's trails would consider Hop Valley to be a particularly challenging or dangerous hike. The trail meanders from the Kolob Terrace Road through an open valley, providing expansive views of the canyon walls and crimson cliffs that bring people from all over the world to see this park. As it continues through the canyon, the trail descends until high walls rise on both sides of hikers. This trail can provide one of the most satisfying wilderness hikes in the park, but it requires no scrambling, climbing, canyoneering, wading, or major ascents.

That's why it's hard to understand what exactly happened to Corey Buxton, a seventeen-year-old Eagle Scout from Las Vegas, on July 22, 2010, when he collapsed, apparently rolled down into a brushy part of the canyon, and lost his life.

Buxton had accompanied his Scout troop to Zion for a four-day hiking and camping adventure. On the second day, the six-foot-three, 230-pound boy began to struggle with the challenge and the heat, and told his Scout leader to "leave him alone," according to the park's incident report. The leader told rangers later than he hiked ahead about one hundred yards and turned around to look for Corey to see if he had followed. Corey was gone.

It took a park search team until the next day to find the boy, using search and rescue dogs to track his whereabouts.

His body finally emerged in a patch of thick brush in a ravine about 225 feet from the trail.

What had gone wrong? The diagnosis was hyperthermia, a prolonged spike in body temperature beyond what a human being can safely tolerate. Buxton had hiked many trails in Zion before and even completed a Boy Scout badge in wilderness survival. The young man may have become too compromised to recognize the warning signs his own body presented—and as part of a troop and as an Eagle Scout to boot, Buxton may have felt that he had to continue beyond his ability to do so.

"On the rare occasion that something like this happens we all hurt together, we all bond together, and eventually we'll do our best to figure out what happened and make sure that we do our best to figure out if there's something that happened that we need to change," said local Boy Scouts of America executive Phil Bevins in a television interview after Buxton was found. "We take that very seriously."

With this story of a high school senior meeting a tragic end, we have now revisited the deaths of all ninety-two people who have perished in Zion National Park to date in the twentieth and twenty-first centuries. In the following pages, I offer a collection of common-sense tips to help you make the most of your visit to this park—and to keep you safe while you do so. Please follow this advice, heed the warnings, and make these simple rules part of every outing as you hike, climb, rappel, wade, bicycle, or ride the shuttle buses through one of the most extraordinary places on earth.

EPILOGUE: HOW TO STAY ALIVE
IN ZION NATIONAL PARK

Are you ready to make the commitment to seeing the best of Zion National Park—its canyons, pools, hanging gardens, rivers, peaks, wildflowers, animals, and clear skies—and living to tell the tale?

It's easier than you may think after reading this book, so let me remind you again: On average, only one to two people per year actually die in the park, and some years no one dies at all. By following a few simple rules and taking some entirely reasonable precautions, you can make the most of your visit and come home with plenty of photos and accounts of your adventures.

Here are the basic guidelines you need, based on the advice of the National Park Service, Zion park management, and experts in hiking and climbing safety. These also apply to just about any park in the system, so keep these general rules in mind no matter where you travel.

AROUND THE PARK

- **Stay on designated trails.** Most people are not prepared to venture off-trail into the backcountry, and you can see plenty of marvelous sights from the established trails throughout the park. Note the directions you'll see on trail signs, and pay attention to blazes and markers to be sure you're still on your intended trail.

- **Stay behind protective fences, guardrails, and barriers.** Barriers are placed for your protection, *not* to keep you from enjoying the park. The moment you step beyond a guardrail or boundary, you risk injury.

- **Watch out for traffic.** When you stop at a pull-off along the side of a road, keep an eye out for oncoming traffic and fast-moving vehicles, just as you would on any busy street. Drivers gazing out over a spectacular view may not see you on the road, so watch out for people who are not watching out for you.

- **If you're driving, watch the road.** It's easy to be distracted by everything there is to see at Zion, so if you want more time to enjoy a view, pull over into an area designated for that purpose and stop. Pedestrians and bicyclists are everywhere along the park's major roadways—so keep an eye out.

Hiking—Frontcountry or Backcountry

- **Don't hike alone.** The lure of solitude in the wild may be very attractive, but a lone hiker who becomes lost or suffers an injury may be missing for weeks, months, or even indefinitely. Hiking and camping with at least one other person can make the difference between a great day on the trail and a misadventure that ends in tragedy.

- **File your plan with a ranger.** If you're planning a lengthy wilderness hike or a canyon exploration or climb, you will need a backcountry permit—which means that you will file a hiking or climbing plan at a ranger station or visitor center. Even if you don't plan to camp, it's a good idea to let rangers know where you intend to go. With thousands of acres of land to search, rangers will depend on the plan you file to narrow the field quickly if they need to locate you in a crisis. Your plan also gives rangers an idea of when you expect to return—so they will know when to start looking for you.

- **Listen to rangers.** People who work in the park daily know which trails may be compromised by weather events, where flash floods and rockslides are possible, where forest fires are burning within the park, and whether it's advisable to attempt the hike or climb you have in mind. If they warn you not to take a certain route, think very seriously about changing your plans.

- **Sign the trail registry.** It may seem like a folksy tradition, but your signature in the trail registry can save your life. It helps rangers discover exactly where you started your hike, so they can narrow a search if you become lost in the wilderness. Hikers who took the same trail in the last few days also may make note of unusual obstacles like rockslides, washed-out stream crossings, or icy areas. Take heed of these warnings as you plan your route.

- **Carry more than you need.** Survival can become critical in the wilderness, so at the very least, bring extra food, clothing, ways to keep warm, and a way to signal your location. Many hiking associations have their own list of the Ten Essentials you should bring on any hike, but here is the most widely accepted classic list:

- Map
- Compass (or other navigation tool, like a GPS)
- Sunglasses and sunscreen
- Extra clothing, including rain gear
- Headlamp or flashlight
- First-aid supplies
- Firestarter—material that will ignite quickly and burn long enough for you to get a fire started
- Matches
- Knife
- Extra food and water

In addition, many hiking clubs recommend that you bring emergency shelter, a repair kit and tools (including a roll of duct tape), and a water filter kit. If you need to signal your location, a mirror can be invaluable.

- **Bring water treatment tools.** Water in the Zion wilderness is not safe to drink without treatment.

  - At the very least, bring water to a rolling boil and allow it to boil for one minute for every thousand feet you are above sea level.

  - Bring an absolute one-micron filter, or one labeled as meeting ANSI/NSF International Standard #53. This will help remove waterborne parasites.

- When you've filtered the water, add eight drops of liquid chlorine bleach or four drops of iodine, and let it stand for thirty minutes before drinking it.

- **Know your limits.** Many hikers and climbers come to Zion to take on a greater challenge than they have ever tried before. If you're one of these adventurers, be sure that you understand the kinds of skills required to complete the climb or canyon successfully. Hike or climb with someone who has the requisite experience to be sure your party gets home safely, and take all the necessary precautions, from carrying the right gear to recognizing that the challenge may be too great.

- **Watch out for slickrock and loose sand.** Zion is a sandstone park, so ledges and slopes can be covered in sand that creates a slippery surface under your feet. Step carefully and gauge the stability of a surface before you tread there, especially if you're walking along narrow ledges. Many climbing and hiking accidents result from unstable rock underfoot.

- **Stay back from cliff edges.** Falls from Emerald Pools, Angels Landing, Canyon Overlook, and other places in the park have resulted in deaths. Most cliff edges in the park have no railings or fences, so it's up to you to take responsibility for your own safety. Edges may be slippery when wet or covered with slippery sand when dry. Observe posted warnings, stay on the trail, and keep a careful eye on your children.

Desert Conditions

Zion is a desert park, so assume you will need at least one gallon of water per person per day on any hike. You can fill your water bottles at any visitor center or campground, and at Zion Lodge.

- **Remember to drink your water as you hike.** You're working hard when you hike, so you're losing hydration as you perspire and even as you breathe harder. Make sure you take in enough water to replace these losses, to maintain a good hydration level. Don't wait until you are thirsty; just keep drinking.

- **Eat salty snacks.** Bring and eat nuts, pretzels, jerky, or your favorite source of salt. This will help you maintain your hydration level.

- **Wear sun protection.** A hat protects your head from the hot sun, and a water-soaked bandana around your neck can help lower your overall body temperature.

- **Know the signs of heat exhaustion.** When your body loses more fluid than it takes in, you can develop heat exhaustion. This is a dangerous condition that requires immediate attention. Signs include nausea, vomiting, fatigue, headaches, pallor, stomach cramps, and skin that feels clammy. Stop hiking and find a cool, shady area to rest, and put your feet up to help redistribute fluids. Drink fluids and eat something—trail mix or another snack with salt will help return your body's chemistry to normal. If two hours pass and you do not feel better, seek medical attention.

- **Know the signs of heat stroke.** If the person with heat exhaustion becomes confused or disoriented, has strange changes in behavior, or actually has a seizure, he or she has progressed to an advanced stage of heat exhaustion known as heat stroke. Cool this person using any means available, and seek help immediately.

On and Around Water

Drowning in a flash flood is a leading cause of death in Zion. Take some basic precautions to keep yourself safe in slot canyons, especially in July and August.

- **Check for flash flood advisories.** Check the National Weather Service online when you plan your canyoneering adventure or your hike through the Narrows, and talk with rangers shortly before you set out. Weather can change suddenly and with little warning, so err on the side of caution. If there's a thunderstorm brewing to the north and you're planning to explore a slot canyon, postpone your plans until the forecast is clear.

- **Watch for indication of a possible flash flood.** Zion National Park lists these signs that a flood may be imminent:
  - Any deterioration in weather conditions
  - A buildup of clouds
  - Thunder
  - Floating debris

- Rising water levels or stronger currents
- Increasing roar of water upcanyon

If you see or hear any of these signs, seek higher ground right away—getting even a few feet higher can save your life. Stay on the high ground until water levels recede.

- **Be prepared to wait out a flash flood.** It can take twenty-four hours or more for flood waters to go down, so be sure to pack extra food, water, and a way to keep warm any time you venture into a narrow canyon.

- **Learn to recognize hypothermia.** When the body cools to a dangerous level, your life can be in danger—and you may not even know it's happening. If you're soaked through from hiking up a narrow canyon, you may not realize that immersion in water is the fastest route to body heat loss. The Zion National Park website lists these symptoms of hypothermia:
  - Uncontrollable shivering
  - Stumbling and poor coordination
  - Fatigue and weakness
  - Confusion or slurred speech

If you develop any of these symptoms, stop hiking and change out of your wet clothing. Never wear cotton clothes while hiking in a narrow canyon, as cotton provides no insulation when it's wet, and it takes a long time to dry, leaving you chilled for a long period.

Eating high-energy food before you get chilled can help you maintain body heat.

- **Stay off of slippery or moss-covered rocks and logs.** It may look like fun to hop from one boulder to the next in the middle of a rushing stream, but you will be surprised at how slick these rocks become when they're wet. Many deaths result from people slipping and falling from these rocks into frigid water.

- **Don't wade into a stream at the top of a waterfall.** It's hard to believe that this needs to be said, but people have died in Zion and other parks (most famously Yosemite) because they wade out into a rushing stream to get a photo of a waterfall from the top. Here's a lifesaving tip from my husband and me, the author and photographer of the book *Hiking Waterfalls in New York*: There's nothing to see up there at the top of the falls. You'll get a much better photo from the bottom—and from the shore.

WILDLIFE

You will encounter animals in Zion, most of which have little if any interest in interacting with you. Wild animals can be unpredictable, however, so follow these simple guidelines to make the most of your sightings safely.

- **Enjoy wildlife from a safe distance.** While no one has died in Zion because of an encounter with an animal, other parks have had their share of deadly encounters, so do not approach any animal you see. To get great photos, shoot with a telephoto lens from a safe distance. If you're in your car and you spot wildlife from the road, pull over at the first available area and take your photos from inside your car.

- **Report sick or injured animals to rangers.** Do not attempt to approach or help an injured animal. A wounded animal may be frightened and will try to defend itself, which will not end well for you. Note the location of the animal and report it to a ranger as soon as you can.

- **Keep an eye out for mountain lions.** Zion has never had a report of a mountain lion attack on a person or pet, but lions have been sighted in the park—and other parks and wilderness areas have records of attacks.

  - Do not allow your children to run ahead or lag behind you on a trail.

  - Don't hike alone; you are more vulnerable to attacks when you are a solo hiker.

  - Do not approach a mountain lion; leave it an escape route so it can pass by without incident.

  - Do not run. Hold your arms above your head and try to look large.

  - If the lion approaches, make noise—shout and throw rocks. Wave your arms to help you look threatening.

- If you are attacked, fight back with all of your strength.
- Above all, do not feed any wildlife in the park.

Follow these guidelines to make your visit to Zion National Park the experience of a lifetime you hope it will be. Once again, I urge you to join more than 3.7 million people who discover and explore this park every year, with the knowledge that a few simple precautions will help you make certain that your trip is memorable for all the right reasons: the outdoor adventures, the wildlife sightings, and the magnificent canyons you will find here in Utah's Grand Circle.

APPENDIX: LIST OF DEATHS 1908–2016
IN CHRONOLOGICAL ORDER

NAME	AGE	DATE OF DEATH	CAUSE	LOCATION
Hepworth, Thornton	About 9	July 28, 1908	Lightning strike	Cable Mountain
Stout, Lionel	About 9	July 28, 1908	Lightning strike	Cable Mountain
Winder, Ether	20	December 18, 1921	Fire	Cable Mountain
McClain, Allan T.	35	January 19, 1928	Construction accident; crushed by a rock	Zion–Mt. Carmel Tunnel
Morrison, Johnny	25	July 1, 1928	Construction accident; breathing in dust, sand, and dynamite	Zion–Mt. Carmel Tunnel
Brooksby, Albin	35	April 11, 1930	Cable accident (falling object)	Cable Mountain
Cafferata, Eugene	19	July 8, 1930	Fell off a 55-foot-high cliff	Lady Mountain
Orcutt, Don	24	July 28, 1931	Climbing accident	Cathedral Mountain
Hirschi, Clair L.	22	August 22, 1937	Motorcycle accident	Zion Park highway near museum
Tanner, Ray	18	February 8, 1938	Blasting accident; died of infection six weeks later	Bridge Mountain CCC camp
Callahan, Evelyn Frances	23	July 1, 1947	Suicide	Emerald Pools trail
Cottrell, Lane Kelton	17	September 4, 1951	Fell from a cliff	Great White Throne area
Bergemeyer, Frederick E.	39	August 23, 1952	Truck accident	On a park trail north and east of the entrance
Long, Mrs. Milo D.	41	August 26, 1958	Fell	Zion–Mt. Carmel Tunnel (gallery window)
Hilton, Kelly	17	August 5, 1959	Fell off a cliff	Trail to Natural Bridge Canyon
Florence, Steven	13	September 17, 1961	Drowned, flash flood	Narrows of the Virgin River

NAME	AGE	DATE OF DEATH	CAUSE	LOCATION
Johnson, Frank	17	September 17, 1961	Drowned, flash flood	Narrows of the Virgin River
Nelson, Alvin	17	September 17, 1961	Drowned, flash flood	Narrows of the Virgin River
Nichols, Ray	17	September 17, 1961	Drowned, flash flood	Narrows of the Virgin River
Scott, Walter	48	September 17, 1961	Drowned, flash flood	Narrows of the Virgin River
Harrison, Dana	11	June 22, 1962	Fell from a cliff	Lady Mountain
Hillery, Ronald	15	October 10, 1965	Climbing accident	Lodge Canyon
Newman, Jean Helen	37	July 23, 1967	Auto accident	Utah 15 (now Utah 9)
Newman, John W.	46	July 23, 1967	Auto accident	Utah 15 (now Utah 9)
Casalou, Robert	13	March 3, 1968	Fell at Upper Pool	Emerald Pools trail
Chin, Norman	54	September 22, 1969	Fell	East Rim Trail
Michael Rose, Steven	21	June 6, 1972	Motorcycle accident	Zion–Mt. Carmel Tunnel
Miller, Steven Lee	26	August 9, 1973	Fell from a cliff	Unnamed cliff
Hoff, Harvey Frank	29	May 26, 1974	Motorcycle accident	Inside a tunnel
Bourne, David	20	March 16, 1978	Fell	Observation Point
Brereton, Thomas	42	April 13, 1979	Fell when a rock broke	West Temple
Russell, John	19	October 16, 1983	Fell from Middle Emerald Pool	Emerald Pools trail
Cooke, James F.	35	April 13, 1986	Bicycle accident	Zion–Mt. Carmel Tunnel
Campbell, Glen	23	November 6, 1987	Plane crash	Northern edge of park
Keller, Michelle	24	November 6, 1987	Plane crash	Northern edge of park
Woolsey, Brad	24	November 6, 1987	Plane crash	Northern edge of park
Dwyer, Jeffrey Robert	28	April 2, 1989	Fell, possible suicide	Angels Landing
Bryant, David Faulkner	32	October 13, 1992	Rappelling accident	Subway (Left Fork of North Creek)
Phillips, Affin William	21	May 13, 1993	Fell, hiking alone	Taylor Creek
Ellis, Kim	37	July 15, 1993	Drowned	Kolob Creek
Fleischer, David Gary	28	July 15, 1993	Drowned	Kolob Creek
Dyer, Marco	29	July 16, 1994	Motorcycle accident	Zion–Mt. Carmel Tunnel
Price, Larry	35	November 22, 1994	Fell	Court of the Patriarchs
Christensen, John Michael	36	January 1, 1997	Rappelling accident	Angels Landing

NAME	AGE	DATE OF DEATH	CAUSE	LOCATION
Eggertz, Tyler Jeffrey	12	March 28, 1997	Fell down a waterfall	Middle Emerald Pool
Bottarini, Patricia	36	May 9, 1997	Fell, husband acquitted of homicide	East Rim Observation Point
Algan, Ramsey E.	27	July 27, 1998	Drowned	Narrows of the Virgin River
Garcia, Paul	31	July 27, 1998	Drowned	Narrows of the Virgin River
Tuell, Shawn	27	August 1, 1998	Fell off slickrock	Hidden Canyon
Simpson, Sasha	20	January 21, 1999	Fell while rappelling	Lodge Canyon
Sender, Georg	63	August 2, 2000	Fell	Angels Landing
Muñoz, Michael	10	May 10, 2001	Fell, flash flood	Canyon Overlook Trail (Pine Creek Canyon)
Lewis, Penny	37	May 16, 2001	Fell, hiking alone	Subway (Left Fork of North Creek)
Tamin, Roselan	35	May 21, 2002	Climbing accident	Spaceshot
Kaiser, Dorothy	66	January 19, 2003	Fell, hiking alone; possible suicide	Scout Lookout
Frankewicz, Christopher	37	September 5, 2003	Climbing accident	Behunin Canyon
Goebel, John	23	March 16, 2004	Accident resulting from drunkenness	Virgin River
Morrow, Colin Robert	21	March 28, 2004	Motorcycle accident	Zion–Mt. Carmel Tunnel
Padilla, Aaron J.	21	March 28, 2004	Motorcycle accident	Zion–Mt. Carmel Tunnel
Jones, Kristoffer	14	June 25, 2004	Fell off a cliff	Angels Landing
Vander Meer, Bernadette	29	August 22, 2006	Hiking accident	Angels Landing
Biedermann, Keith	48	June 4, 2007	Fell while rappelling	Heaps Canyon
Goldstein, Barry S.	53	June 8, 2007	Hiking accident	Angels Landing
Ertischek, Mark	60	June 9, 2007	Heart attack	Angels Landing
Welton, James Martin	34	October 17, 2008	Climbing accident	Touchstone
Forster, Craig	55	November 28, 2008	Fell	Unnamed side canyon off Utah 9
Brigham, David	48	February 25, 2009	Suicide	Canyon Overlook
Maltez, Nancy	55	August 9, 2009	Hiking accident	Angels Landing
Grunig, Tammy	50	November 27, 2009	Hiking accident	Angels Landing
Chidester, Daniel	23	April 25, 2010	Drowned	Narrows of the Virgin River

Appendix

NAME	AGE	DATE OF DEATH	CAUSE	LOCATION
Scaffidi, Jesse	23	April 25, 2010	Drowned	Narrows of the Virgin River
Milobedzki, Regine	63	April 27, 2010	Fell, hiking alone	Scout Lookout
Buxton, Corey	17	July 22, 2010	Hyperthermia	Hop Valley Trail
Hosobuchi, Yoshio	74	September 18, 2012	Canyoneering accident	Subway (Left Fork of North Creek)
Hurd III, Lyle David	49	October 26, 2012	Climbing accident	Northeast Buttress (below Angels Landing)
Schena, Scott	22	July 20, 2013	Climbing accident	Employee Falls
Johnson, Karen	51	July 26, 2013	Model T flipped over	Utah 9, just outside the park
Haas, Cheri	47	September 5, 2013	Canyoneering accident	Subway (Left Fork of North Creek)
Bellows, Amber	28	February 8, 2014	BASE jumping accident	Mount Kinesava
Leary, Sean	38	March 13, 2014	BASE jumping accident	Three Marys (West Temple area)
Yoshi Vo, Douglas	34	September 27, 2014	Drowned	Narrows of the Virgin River
Spencer, Christopher	47	October 19, 2014	Climbing accident	Iron Messiah route
Artmann, Bryan	24	July 12, 2015	Canyoneering accident	Heaps Canyon
Arthur, Linda	57	September 14, 2015	Drowned, flash flood	Keyhole Canyon
Arthur, Steve	58	September 14, 2015	Drowned, flash flood	Keyhole Canyon
Brum, Robin	53	September 14, 2015	Drowned, flash flood	Keyhole Canyon
Favela, Gary	51	September 14, 2015	Drowned, flash flood	Keyhole Canyon
MacKenzie, Mark	56	September 14, 2015	Drowned, flash flood	Keyhole Canyon
Reynolds, Muku	59	September 14, 2015	Drowned, flash flood	Keyhole Canyon
Teichner, Don	55	September 14, 2015	Drowned, flash flood	Keyhole Canyon
Johnson, Christian Louis	50	October 2, 2015	Rappelling accident	Not Imlay Canyon
Klimt, Eric Michael	36	March 9, 2016	Climbing accident	Moonlight Buttress

BIBLIOGRAPHY

CHAPTER 1

Associated Press. "Zion National Park Hiker, Douglas Yoshi Vo, Killed by Flooding at Utah Park, Authorities Say." Weather.com, September 30, 2014. Accessed July 29, 2016. https://weather.com/travel/news/zion -national-park-flooding-hiker-dies-20140930.

"Bodies Found in Zion Identified." National Park Service news release, April 28, 2010. Accessed July 29, 2016. www.nps.gov/zion/learn/news/ bodies-found-in-zion-identified.htm.

"Body Found in Zion National Park." National Park Service news release, April 26, 2010. Accessed July 29, 2016. www.nps.gov/zion/learn/news/ body-found-in-zion-national-park.htm.

Braun, Joe. "The Zion Narrows." Joe's Guide to Zion National Park. Accessed July 29, 2016. www.citrusmilo.com/zionguide/zionnarrows.cfm.

"Crew of 200 Joins Hunt for 2 Hikers." *Ogden Standard-Examiner*, September 23, 1961. Accessed July 28, 2016. www.newspapers.com/ image/14216820/?terms=Alvin%2BNelson.

"Current Conditions." Zion National Park website. Accessed July 29, 2016. www.nps.gov/zion/planyourvisit/conditions.htm.

"Death Toll May Reach Five in Zion Park Flood." *Daily Herald* (Provo, UT), September 19, 1961. Accessed July 28, 2016. www.newspapers.com/ image/25619807/?terms=%22Zion%2BNational%2BPark%22%2Bdeath.

"Flash Flood–Refrigerator Canyon." Climb-Utah.com. Accessed July 25, 2016. www.climb-utah.com/Zion/flash_zion.htm.

Foy, Paul. "Rafters Killed in Zion National Park Identified." KSL.com, April 27, 2010. Accessed July 29, 2016. https://www.ksl.com/?sid=10550591.

"Hikers Find Body Floating in Virgin River." *Salt Lake Tribune*, July 29, 1998, as reposted on Climb-Utah.com. Accessed July 25, 2016. www.climb -utah.com/Zion/flash_zion.htm.

Jensen, Frank. "Hike Leader Paints Picture of Tragedy." *Salt Lake Tribune*, September 19, 1961. Accessed July 28, 2016. www.newspapers.com/ image/9846436.

———. "S. Utah Flood Kills 3 from S.L. Area." *Salt Lake Tribune*, September 19, 1961. Accessed July 28, 2016. www.newspapers.com/ image/9846386/?terms=Alvin%2BNelson.

Knoss, Trent. "Hiker Dies in Zion Narrows." Backpacker.com. Accessed July 29, 2016. www.backpacker.com/news-and-events/news/trail-news/hiker-dies-in-zion-narrows.

Mahoney, Sean. "Zion National Park: Hiker Perishes after Getting Stuck in Flooded 'Narrows.'" Inquisitr.com, September 29, 2014. Accessed July 29, 2016. www.inquisitr.com/1507920/zion-national-park-hiker-perishes-after-getting-stuck-in-flooded-narrows.

McFall, Michael, and Wendy Ogata. "Utah Forecast: Rainfall Sets Records, Another Storm on Its Way." *Salt Lake Tribune*, September 28, 2014. Accessed July 29, 2016. www.sltrib.com/sltrib/news/58464984-78/inches-state-according-county.html.csp.

"Narrows Victim Identified." National Park Service news release, July 29, 1998, as reposted on Climb-Utah.com. Accessed July 25, 2016. www.climb-utah.com/Zion/flash_zion.htm.

"No More Organized Searching Is Planned . . ." *Daily Herald* (Provo, UT), September 25, 1961. Accessed July 28, 2016. www.newspapers.com/image/25621372/?terms=Alvin%2BNelson.

"Parents of Two Missing Hikers Remain at Scene of Zion National Park Flash Flood." *Daily Herald* (Provo, UT), September 20, 1961. Accessed July 28, 2016. www.newspapers.com/image/25620172.

"Remembering Douglass Yoshi Vo." YouCaring.com, October 1, 2014. Accessed July 29, 2016. www.youcaring.com/memorial-fundraiser/remembering-the-douglass-yoshi-vo/241463.

"Search for Two Missing Hikers to Be Intensified." *Daily Herald* (Provo, UT), September 21, 1961. Accessed July 28, 2016. www.newspapers.com/image/25620540.

"Searchers Find Second Body in Zion National Park." National Park Service news release, April 27, 2010. Accessed July 29, 2016. www.nps.gov/zion/learn/news/searchers-find-second-body-in-zion-national-park.htm.

"Second Body Pulled from Virgin River." *Salt Lake Tribune*, July 30, 1998, as reposted on Climb-Utah.com. Accessed July 25, 2016. www.climb-utah.com/Zion/flash_zion.htm.

Sheer, Julie. "More Deaths at Zion National Park." Outposts, *Los Angeles Times*, April 28, 2010. Accessed July 29, 2016. http://latimesblogs.latimes.com/outposts/2010/04/another-death-at-angels-landing.html.

Skoloff, Brian. "Skull Linked to UT Scout Missing Since 1961 Flood." *San Diego Union-Tribune*, May 11, 2012. Accessed July 28, 2016. www.sandiegouniontribune.com/news/2012/may/11/skull-linked-to-ut-scout-missing-since-1961-flood/.

"What is a Cubic Foot Per Second?" Boulder Area Sustainability Information Network. Accessed July 29, 2016. http://bcn.boulder.co.us/basin/watershed/cubicfeetpersecond.html.

Young, Spencer, and Joe Bauman. "One Dead, One Missing in Zion Park Flash Floods." *Deseret News*, July 29, 1998. Accessed July 27, 2016.

www.deseretnews.com/article/643900/One-dead-one-missing-in-Zion
-Park-flash-floods.html?pg=all.

Chapter 2

Associated Press. "Zion National Park Investigates September's Flash Flood–
Related Deaths." *St. George News*, October 6, 2015. Accessed August 3,
2016. www.stgeorgeutah.com/news/archive/2015/10/06/apc-zion
-national-park-investigates-septembers-flash-flood-related-deaths.

Boyle, Darren. "Pictured: The Seven Hikers Swept to Their Deaths in Utah
Flash Floods—Despite Being Warned about the Danger Hours Before."
MailOnline, *Daily Mail*, September 17, 2015. Accessed August 3, 2016.
www.dailymail.co.uk/news/article-3239397/Body-seventh-hiker-Zion
-National-Park-Utah.html.

Burrows, Shane. "Flash Death?" Canyon Collective discussion forum, May 15,
2001. Accessed August 4, 2016. http://canyoncollective.com/threads/
flash-death.1631.

DeMille, David. "Zion Flood Deaths a Reminder of Wilderness Dangers." *Spectrum* (St. George, UT), September 26, 2015. Accessed
August 3, 2016. www.thespectrum.com/story/news/2015/09/26/
zion-flood-deaths-reminder-wilderness-dangers/72882518.

"Flashflood–Refrigerator Canyon." Climb-Utah.com. Accessed August 4, 2016.
www.climb-utah.com/Zion/flash_zion.htm.

Hanscom, Greg. "Feds Set 'Terrible Precedent' with Kolob Canyon Settlement." *High Country News* (Paonia, CO), August 5, 1996. Accessed
August 2, 2016. www.hcn.org/issues/87/2695.

Jones, Tom. "Kolob Canyon, Zion National Park." CanyoneeringUSA.com.
Accessed August 2, 2016. www.canyoneeringusa.com/utah/zion/
technical/kolob-canyon.

Milligan, Tanya. "Canyon Overlook Trail." ZionNational-Park.com. Accessed
August 4, 2016. www.zionnational-park.com/zion-canyon-overlook-trail
.htm.

Schaffer, Grayson. "Special Report: The Keyhole Seven." *Outside*, May 24,
2016. Accessed August 3, 2016. www.outsideonline.com/2072666/
special-report-keyhole-seven.

Smith, Christopher, and Ray Ring. "Whose Fault? A Utah Canyon Turns
Deadly." *High Country News* (Paonia, CO), August 22, 1994. Accessed
August 2, 2016. www.hcn.org/issues/14/409.

Spangler, Jerry. "He Watched in Horror as Friend Slipped Away." *Deseret
News*, July 22, 1993. Accessed August 1, 2016. https://news.google.com/
newspapers?nid=336&dat=19930722&id=Az9TAAAAIBAJ&sjid=3
YQDAAAAIBAJ&pg=5285,2883537&hl=en.

"Utah Canyoneering History: Morning Reports Excerpts–1994." Canyoneering USA.com. Accessed August 2, 2016. www.canyoneeringusa.com/history/mr1994.htm.

Willis, Clint. "Law: Who's to Blame for Kolob Creek?" *Outside*, May 1994. Accessed August 2, 2016. www.outsideonline.com/1840311/law-whos -blame-kolob-creek.

Yardley, William, Matt Pearce, and Nigel Duara. "Seven Hikers' Descent into Doom at Zion National Park." *Los Angeles Times*, September 20, 2015. Accessed August 2, 2016. http://graphics.latimes.com/zion-flash-flood.

"Young Hiker Who Died at Zion Is Identified." *Deseret News*, May 15, 2001. Accessed August 4, 2016. https://news.google.com/newspapers?nid =336&dat=20010515&id=KwckAAAAIBAJ&sjid=re0DAAAAIBAJ& pg=1756,8095509&hl=en%20%20also%20in%20Zion%20deaths%20 book.

"Zion National Park Releases Names of Keyhole Canyon Fatalities." National Park Service news release, September 17, 2015. Accessed August 3, 2016. www.nps.gov/zion/learn/news/keyholeflashfloodsept17.htm.

Chapter 3

"01-24-2003 Zion National Park (UT) Falling Fatality." Utah Canyoneering History: Morning Reports Excerpts–2003 First Half. Canyoneering USA.com. Accessed August 9, 2016. www.canyoneeringusa.com/history/mr2003a.htm.

Associated Press. "Botched Rappel Blamed in Death of Zion Climber." *Deseret News*, January 22, 1997. Accessed August 9, 2016. http://beta.deseret news.com/article/538873/botched-rappel-blamed-in-death-of-zion -climber.html.

———. "Idaho Man's Death in Park Investigated." *Spokesman-Review*, April 4, 2016. Accessed August 5, 2016. https://news.google.com/newspapers ?nid=1314&dat=19890404&id=m1lWAAAAIBAJ&sjid=xO8DAAAA IBAJ&pg=3054,2588154&hl=en.

———. "Third Death in a Week at Zion National Park." KSL.com, June 11, 2007. Accessed August 9, 2016. www.ksl.com/?nid=148&sid=1331100.

———. "Woman Dead after Fall in Zion National Park." KSL.com, August 22, 2006. Accessed August 10, 2016. www.ksl.com/?nid=148&sid=439979.

"Bernadette Vander Meer." Obituary, *Las Vegas Review-Journal*, August 23, 2006. Accessed August 10, 2016. http://obits.reviewjournal.com/ obituaries/lvrj/obituary.aspx?pid=142067472.

"Bonner County Man's Body Found." *Spokane Chronicle*, April 4, 1989. Accessed August 5, 2016. https://news.google.com/newspapers?nid =1345&dat=19890404&id=-scSAAAAIBAJ&sjid=7fkDAAAAIBAJ& pg=5719,147028&hl=en.

"Boy Falls to Death During Hiking Trip." *Lakeland Ledger*, June 27, 2004. Accessed August 9, 2016. https://news.google.com/newspapers?nid =1346&dat=20040627&id=W_EvAAAAIBAJ&sjid=y_0DAAAAIBAJ &pg=6487,3121013&hl=en.

Burnett, Jim. "Fatal Fall from Angels Landing in Zion National Park." National ParksTraveler.com, August 10, 2009. Accessed August 10, 2016. www .nationalparkstraveler.com/2009/08/fall-angels-landing-zion-national -park-claims-life-california-woman.

"California Teen Dies in Fall at Utah Park." *USA Today*, June 27, 2004. Accessed August 9, 2016. http://usatoday30.usatoday.com/news/ nation/2004-06-27-utah-teen_x.htm.

Chick Tower. "Angels Landing Death." Rec.Backcountry newsgroup, August 2006, found in Narkive (newsgroup archive). Accessed August 10, 2016. http://rec.backcountry.narkive.com/dstd2unF/angels-landing-death.

"Death: John Christensen." *Deseret News*, January 5, 1997. Accessed August 9, 2016. http://beta.deseretnews.com/article/535777/death-john -christensen.html.

DeMasters, Tiffany. "Hiker Collapses, Dies on Zion Trail." *Spectrum* (St. George, UT), June 11, 2007, as posted on the Canyon Collective discussion forum. Accessed August 9, 2016. http://canyoncollective.com/ threads/hiker-collapses-dies-on-zion-trail.11317.

"Dr. Barry Steven Goldstein." FindAGrave.com. Accessed August 10, 2016. www.findagrave.com/cgi-bin/fg.cgi?page=gr&GRid=114827815.

"Falling Fatality from Angels Landing in Zion National Park." National Park Service news release, June 10, 2007. Accessed August 10, 2016. www.nps .gov/zion/learn/news/falling-fatality-from-angels-landing-in-zion -national-park.htm.

"Falling Victim Identified." National Park Service news release, May 4, 2010. Accessed August 12, 2016. www.nps.gov/zion/learn/news/falling-victim -identified.htm.

"Glendora Woman Plunges 1,000 Feet to Death in Utah's Zion National Park." *Los Angeles Times*, August 9, 2009. Accessed August 10, 2016. http://latimesblogs.latimes.com/lanow/2009/08/glendora-woman -plunges-1000-feet-to-death-in-utahs-zion-national-park.html.

Hale, Natalie. "Hiker Plunges from a Trail in Zion Park." *Deseret News*, June 9, 2007. Accessed August 10, 2016. http://beta.deseretnews.com/article/ 660228165/Hiker-plunges-from-a-trail-in-Zion-Park.html?pg=all.

Haraden, Tom. "00-456–Zion NP (UT)–Falling Fatality." Morning Report Canyoneering Excerpts Year 2000. CanyoneeringUSA.com. Accessed August 9, 2016. www.canyoneeringusa.com/mag/safety/mcan00.htm.

Jones, Tom. "Angels Landing, Zion National Park." CanyoneeringUSA.com. Accessed August 9, 2016. www.canyoneeringusa.com/utah/zion/trails/ angels-landing-zion-national-park.

LaPlante, Matthew D. "A Deadly Wager." *Salt Lake Tribune*, September 4, 2004. Accessed August 9, 2016. http://archive.sltrib.com/story.php?ref=/ci_2407635.

Neff, Elizabeth. "Mom Sues over Scout's Fall Off Cliff." *Salt Lake Tribune*, June 14, 2006. Accessed August 9, 2016. http://archive.sltrib.com/story.php?ref=/utah/ci_3934362.

"Once Infamous, Angels Landing Trail Now a Safety Success Story." *Salt Lake Tribune*, June 14, 2015. Accessed August 12, 2016. www.sltrib.com/blogs/hiking/2558551-155/once-infamous-angels-landing-trail-now.

"Preliminary Autopsy Shows No Sign of Foul Play in Death of Zion Hiker but Park Service Officials, FBI Are Still Labeling Case as 'Suspicious.'" *Deseret News*, April 5, 1989. Accessed August 5, 2016. www.deseretnews.com/article/41031/preliminary-autopsy-shows-no-sign-of-foul-play-in-death-of-zion-hiker.html.

Ranaivo, Yann. "Local Woman Dies in Fall in Zion National Park." *Idaho State Journal*, November 29, 2009. Accessed August 12, 2016. http://idahostatejournal.com/local-woman-dies-in-fall-in-zion-national-park/article_026646cc-dcbd-11de-a56e-001cc4c03286.html.

Repanshek, Kurt. "Woman Dies in Fall from Angels Landing." NationalParks Traveler.com, August 23, 2006. Accessed August 10, 2016. www.nationalparkstraveler.com/2006/08/woman-dies-fall-angels-landing.

Rogers, Melinda. "Zion National Park Records Third Fatality in a Week." *Salt Lake Tribune*, April 29, 2010. Accessed August 12, 2016. www.lowellsun.com/police/ci_14975623.

Sheer, Julie. "Angels Landing Dangers." Outposts, *Los Angeles Times*, August 10, 2009. Accessed August 12, 2016. http://latimesblogs.latimes.com/outposts/2009/08/angels-landing-dangers.html.

———. "Angels Landing Update." Outposts, *Los Angeles Times*, August 13, 2009. Accessed August 12, 2016. http://latimesblogs.latimes.com/outposts/2009/08/angels-landing-update-1.html.

St. Germain, Patrice. "Zion National Park Has First Fatality in 2 Years." *Spectrum* (St. George, UT), August 23, 2006, as posted on the Canyon Collective discussion forum. Accessed August 10, 2016. http://canyoncollective.com/threads/fall-from-angels-landing.9924.

United Press International. "Death of Zion Hiker Probed." *Deseret News*, April 4, 2016. Accessed August 5, 2016. https://news.google.com/newspapers?nid=2318&dat=19890404&id=wo0pAAAAIBAJ&sjid=O4QDAAAAIBAJ&pg=2656,1574268&hl=en.

"When Things Go Wrong on the Trail: Four Cases Show How Scout Outings Can Turn Deadly." *Los Angeles Times*, December 5, 2010. Accessed August 9, 2016. http://articles.latimes.com/2010/dec/05/nation/la-na-scouts-box-20101205.

Winslow, Ben. "Fatal Fall at Zion Is Investigated." *Deseret News*, August 23, 2006. Accessed August 10, 2016. http://beta.deseretnews.com/article/645195423/Fatal-fall-at-Zion-is-investigated.html.

"Woman Falls from Angels Landing in Zion National Park." National Park Service news release, November 30, 2009. Accessed August 12, 2016. www.nps.gov/zion/learn/news/woman-falls-from-angels-landing-in-zion-national-park.htm.

CHAPTER 4

"01-223–Zion NP (UT)–Possible Falling Fatality." Utah Canyoneering History: Morning Report Excerpts–2001 First Half, CanyoneeringUSA.com. Accessed August 16, 2016. www.canyoneeringusa.com/history/mr2001a.htm.

"11-Year-Old Son of Mr. and Mrs. Thede Harrison Is Killed in Fall." *Star Valley Independent*, June 28, 1962, as reposted on FindaGrave.com. Accessed August 14, 2016. www.findagrave.com/cgi-bin/fg.cgi?page=gr&GRid=74186502.

"Affin William Phillips." Highland High School Class of 1990. Accessed August 14, 2016. www.highland1990.com/class_inmemory.cfm.

Associated Press. "1,200-Foot Fall Kills Visitor." *Idaho State Journal*, September 28, 1969. Accessed August 14, 2016. www.newspapers.com/clip/5738507/idaho_state_journal.

———. "Hiker Who Fell off Cliff Was S.L. Man." *Deseret News*, May 18, 1993. Accessed August 14, 2016. http://beta.deseretnews.com/article/291014/hiker-who-fell-off-cliff-was-SL-man.html.

———. "Lafayette Student Killed in Fall in Utah." *Courier-Journal*, March 19, 1978. Accessed August 14, 2016. www.newspapers.com/image/?spot=5739323.

———. "Suits Target Safety in US Parks." *Eugene Register-Guard*, February 12, 2000. Accessed August 15, 2016. https://news.google.com/newspapers?nid=1310&dat=20000212&id=MvRYAAAAIBAJ&sjid=-OsDAAAAIBAJ&pg=5936,2937928&hl=en.

———. "Youth Falls 125 Feet to Death." *Abilene Reporter-News*, August 6, 1959. Accessed August 14, 2016. www.newspapers.com/image/45229547/?terms=death%2Bzion%2Bnational%2Bpark.

Braun, Joe. "Hidden Canyon." Joe's Guide to Zion National Park. Accessed August 15, 2016. www.citrusmilo.com/zionguide/hiddencanyon.cfm.

"Canyon Fall in S. Utah Claims Teen." *Salt Lake Tribune*, March 5, 1968. Accessed August 14, 2016. www.newspapers.com/clip/5738483/the_salt_lake_tribune.

"Colorado Man Dies after Fall off Slickrock in Zion Park." *Deseret News*, August 4, 1998. Accessed August 15, 2016. http://beta.deseretnews.com/

article/644888/Colorado-man-dies-after-fall-off-slickrock-in-Zion-Park
.html.

"Coloradoan Falls to Death in Zion National Park." *Deseret News,* November
24, 1994. Accessed August 15, 2016. http://beta.deseretnews
.com/article/389463/coloradan-falls-to-death-in-zion-national-park.html.

"Dana O. Harrison." FindaGrave.com. Accessed August 14, 2016. www
.findagrave.com/cgi-bin/fg.cgi?page=gr&GRid=74186502.

"Fall Is Fatal to Ex-Louisvillian." *Courier-Journal* (Louisville, KY), August
11, 1973. Accessed August 14, 2016. www.newspapers.com/image/
110184786/?terms=Steven%2BLee%2BMiller.

"Fullerton Man Found Dead in Zion Park." *Independent Press-Telegram* (Long
Beach, CA), September 28, 1969. Accessed August 14, 2016. www
.newspapers.com/clip/5738584/independent_presstelegram.

Jensen, Frank. "Zion Park Fall Kills Murray Youth." *Salt Lake Tribune,* August
6, 1959. Accessed August 14, 2016. www.newspapers.com/image/
12354128/?terms=Kelly%2BHilton%2Bdeath%2BZion.

Jolley, Faith Heaton. "Worst Rockfalls, Landslides in Zion National Park."
KSL.com, October 24, 2015. Accessed August 14, 2016. www.ksl.com/
?sid=37074368&nid=148.

Jones, Tom. "Lady Mountain, Zion National Park." Tom's Utah Canyoneering
Guide. Accessed August 12, 2016. www.canyoneeringusa.com/utah/zion/
off-trail/lady-mountain.

Milligan, Tanya. "Zion: Lady Mountain." ZionNational-Park.com. Accessed
August 12, 2016. www.zionnational-park.com/zion-lady-mountain
.htm.

Nally, Dave, and Bo Beck. *Flash Floods and Falls, Deaths and Rescues in Zion
National Park.* CreateSpace Independent Publishing, Kindle edition,
2013.

"Name Released of Falling Fatality Victim in Zion National Park." National
Park Service news release, December 1, 2008. Accessed August 16, 2016.
www.nps.gov/zion/learn/news/name-released-of-falling-fatality-victim
-in-zion-national-park.htm.

Nancy Elder and Jeffrey D. Eggertz, Plaintiffs-appellants, v. United States of
America, Defendant-appellee, 312 F.3d 1172 (10th Cir. 2002). Accessed
on Justia.com, August 15, 2016. http://law.justia.com/cases/federal/
appellate-courts/F3/312/1172/608818.

Norlen, Clayton. "Victim of Hiking Fall Was U. Director of Sustainability."
Deseret News, December 1, 2008. Accessed August 16, 2016. http://beta
.deseretnews.com/article/705267177/Victim-of-hiking-fall-was-U
-director-of-sustainability.html?pg=all%20%20%20http://www.ksl.com/
?nid=148&sid=4950914.

"Penny D. Lewis." Obituary, Hansen-Spear Funeral Home. Accessed August
16, 2016. www.hansenspear.com/obituary/penny-d-lewis.

Perkins, Nancy. "Texas Hiker Found Dead in Zion Park." *Deseret News*, May 17, 2001. Accessed August 16, 2016. http://beta.deseretnews.com/article/843189/Texas-hiker-found-dead-in-Zion-Park.html.

"Scott Vincent Schena." Obituary, *Lowell Sun*, January 29, 2014. Accessed August 18, 2016. www.legacy.com/obituaries/lowellsun/obituary.aspx?pid=169390312.

"Service Saturday to Honor Victim of Zion Park Fall." *Salt Lake Tribune*, August 7, 1959. Accessed August 14, 2016. www.newspapers.com/image/12355817/?terms=Kelly%2BHilton%2Bdeath%2BZion.

"St. Louis Youth Killed in Fall on Utah Mountain." *St. Louis Post-Dispatch*, July 11, 1930. Accessed August 12, 2016. www.newspapers.com/image/138904881/?terms=%22Zion%2BNational%2BPark%22%2Bdeath.

"The Summit Fund." Utah State University Department of Geology. Accessed August 16, 2016. http://geology.usu.edu/htm/the-summit-fund.

"Third Fatality in Less Than a Week in ZNP." Canyon Collective discussion forum, April 28, 2010. Accessed August 14, 2016. http://canyoncollective.com/threads/third-fatality-in-less-than-a-week-in-znp.15437.

Toomer, Jennifer. "Sandy Boy Perishes in Fall from Zion Cliff." *Deseret News*, March 30, 1997. Accessed August 15, 2016. http://beta.deseretnews.com/article/551531/Sandy-boy-perishes-in-fall-from-Zion-cliff.html.

United Press International. "Logan Boy, 11, Killed in Fall from Ledge at Zion." *Daily Herald* (Provo, UT), June 22, 1962. Accessed August 14, 2016. www.newspapers.com/clip/5747818/the_daily_herald.

———. "Youth Killed in Canyon Plunge." *Green Bay Press-Gazette*, August 6, 1959. Accessed August 14, 2016. www.newspapers.com/image/188848689/?terms=Kelly%2BHilton%2Bdeath%2BZion.

———. "Youth Killed in Cliff Fall at Zion Park." *Ogden Standard-Examiner*, March 5, 1968. Accessed August 14, 2016. www.newspapers.com/clip/5738462/the_ogden_standardexaminer.

"Utah Canyoneering History: Morning Report Excerpts–1993." Canyoneering USA.com. Accessed August 14, 2016. www.canyoneeringusa.com/history/mr1993.htm.

"Utah Canyoneering History: Morning Report Excerpts–1994." Canyoneering USA.com. Accessed August 15, 2016. www.canyoneeringusa.com/history/mr1994.htm.

"West Temple, III, 5.8." SummitPost.org. Accessed August 14, 2016. www.summitpost.org/west-temple-iii-5-8/286540.

"Youth Killed in Zion Park by Long Fall." *Ogden Standard-Examiner*, July 11, 1930. Accessed August 12, 2016. www.newspapers.com/image/23746969/?terms=%22Zion%2BNational%2BPark%22%2Bdeath.

"Zion National Park (UT): Concession Employee Dies of Injuries Sustained in Fall." National Park Service Morning Report, July 25, 2013, as reposted on SuperTopo.com. Accessed August 18, 2016. www.supertopo.com/ climbing/thread.php?topic_id=1587523&tn=80.

Chapter 5

"1992-555 Zion (UT) SAR; Fatality." Left Fork (The Subway) and Right Fork Accident Reports, CanyoneeringUSA.com. Accessed August 17, 2016. www.canyoneeringusa.com/subway-accident-reports.

Allred, Drew. "Update: Search Teams Locate Body of Zion BASE Jumper." *St. George News*, February 9, 2014. Accessed August 21, 2016. www .stgeorgeutah.com/news/archive/2014/02/09/eda-update-search-teams -locate-body-of-zion-base-jumper/#.V7pQqGXMSq4.

———. "Update: Zion BASE Jumper Went Down Before Husband, Name Released." *St. George News*, February 9, 2014. Accessed August 21, 2016. www.stgeorgeutah.com/news/archive/2014/02/09/eda-zion-base-jumper -went-went-down-before-her-husband/#.V7oArWXMSq5.

Associated Press. "Climber Falls in Zion Park." *Idaho State Journal*, October 11, 1965. Accessed August 16, 2016. www.newspapers.com/clip/5739126/ idaho_state_journal.

———. "Man Dies Hanging Upside Down at Utah's Zion National Park." *Great Falls Tribune*, September 21, 2012. Accessed August 18, 2016. www.newspapers.com/image/127240507/?terms=%22Zion%2BNational %2BPark%22%2Bdeath.

Barrett, Natalie. "News Short: BASE Jumper's Chute Does Not Deploy; Fatal- ity." *St. George News*, February 8, 2014. Accessed August 21, 2016. www .stgeorgeutah.com/news/archive/2014/02/08/nab-news-short-base -jumpers-chute-does-not-deploy-fatality.

"Canyoneer Dies from Fall in Zion's Subway." *St. George News*, September 6, 2013. Accessed August 19, 2016. www.stgeorgeutah.com/news/archive/ 2013/09/06/canyoneer-dies-fall-zions-subway.

"Canyoneering Fatality in Not Imlay Canyon in Zion National Park." National Park Service news release, October 3, 2015. Accessed August 19, 2016. www.nps.gov/zion/learn/news/canyoneeringfatality_notimlay.htm.

Carpenter, Hayden. "Climber Dies in Fall from Moonlight Buttress." *Rock and Ice*, March 14, 2016. Accessed August 20, 2016. www.rockandice.com/ climbing-accidents/climber-dies-in-fall-from-moonlight-buttress-zion.

Carswell, Cally. "Deaths Renew Calls for National Parks to Rescind BASE Jumping Bans." *High Country News*, July 20, 2015. Accessed August 21, 2016. www.hcn.org/issues/47.12/deaths-renew-calls-for-national-parks -to-rescind-base-jumping-bans.

Chawkins, Steve. "Sean 'Stanley' Leary Dies at 38; Mountain Adventurer." *Los Angeles Times*, March 29, 2014. Accessed August 21, 2016. http://articles .latimes.com/2014/mar/29/local/la-me-sean-leary-20140330.

"Climber Dies in Fall at Zion National Park." National Park Service news release, October 27, 2012. Accessed August 18, 2016. www.nps.gov/zion/learn/news/climber-dies-in-fall-at-zion-national-park.htm.

"Climbing Fatality Name Released." National Park Service news release, October 21, 2014. Accessed August 19, 2016. www.nps.gov/zion/learn/news/climbingfatalitynamed.htm.

"Climbing Fatality on Touchstone Route in Zion National Park." National Park Service press release, October 18, 2008. Accessed August 18, 2016. www.nps.gov/zion/learn/news/climbing-fatality-on-touchstone-route -in-zion-national-park.htm.

Connors, Richard. "Death in Zion (and Stuff about Abseil Knots)." uk.rec .climbing, as reposted on the Canyon Collective discussion forum. Accessed on August 17, 2016. http://canyoncollective.com/threads/zion-fatality.3117.

Dowsett, Ben. "1 dead in Zion National Park Canyoneering Accident." KSL.com, October 3, 2015. Accessed August 19, 2016. www.ksl.com/?sid=36799608&nid=148&s_cid=rss-extlink.

"Falls 1000 Feet to Sudden Death in Zion Canyon." *Iron County Record,* July 29, 1931. Accessed August 16, 2016. https://newspapers.lib.utah.edu/details?id=3784235&q=Don+Orcutt+death&eq=&page=1&rows=50& core=udn&fd=title_t%2Cpaper_t%2Cdate_tdt%2Ctype_t#t_3784235.

"Fatality in Heaps." Discussion thread on Bogley.com, started July 12, 2015. Accessed August 19, 2016. www.bogley.com/forum/showthread .php?74568-Fatality-in-Heaps.

"Fatality in Not Imlay Canyon." Zion National Park Search and Rescue blog, April 21, 2016. Accessed August 19, 2016. www.nps.gov/zion/blogs/Fatality-in-Not-Imlay-Canyon.htm.

"Fatality in Zion National Park's Subway." National Park service news release, September 19, 2012. Accessed August 18, 2016. www.nps.gov/zion/learn/news/fatality-in-subway.htm.

Foy, Paul. "Man dies hanging upside down in Utah's Zion park." *Deseret News,* September 20, 2012. Accessed August 18, 2016. http://www.deseretnews .com/article/765605603/Man-dies-hanging-upside-down-at-Utahs -Zion-park.html

GSH. "To Prophesy Wall: A Story of Life, Death, and Climbing." *Southwest Journal,* January 28, 2014 (first published in *Utah Adventure Journal,* Summer 2013). Accessed August 18, 2016. https://thesouthwestjournal .com/2014/01/28/to-prophesy-wall-a-story-of-life-death-climbing.

Hammill, Ryan. "Foul Play Ruled Out in Climber's Death." *Orange County Register,* June 8, 2007. Accessed August 17, 2016. www.ocregister.com/articles/biedermann-177355-park-adams.html.

Hyland, Dallas. "Louis Johnson Was My Friend." *Independent* (St. George, UT), October 4, 2015. Accessed August 19, 2016. http://suindependent .com/louis-johnson.

Jim, Cami Cox. "Authorities Identify Man Killed by 100-Foot Fall in Zion National Park." *St. George News*, July 14, 2015. Accessed August 19, 2016. www.stgeorgeutah.com/news/archive/2015/07/14/ccj-fatal-fall -zion.

Jolley, Faith Heaton. "Worst Rockfalls, Landslides in Zion National Park." KSL.com, October 24, 2015. Accessed August 17, 2016. www.ksl.com/ ?sid=37074368&nid=148.

Jones, Tom. "Heaps Canyon, Zion National Park." Accessed August 17. 2016. http://www.canyoneeringusa.com/utah/zion/technical/preface/heaps/.

"Man Who Fell in Zion ID'd." *Deseret News*, June 7, 2007. Accessed August 17, 2016. http://beta.deseretnews.com/article/660227287/Man-who-fell -in-Zion-IDd.html.

McFall, Michael. "Clayton Butler, Adventurer Whose Wife Died in Utah BASE Jump, Dies in Hawaii Fall." *Salt Lake Tribune*, January 24, 2015. Accessed August 21, 2016. www.sltrib.com/lifestyle/outdoors/2072592 -155/clayton-butler-adventurer-whose-wife.

Meek, Doug. "Icewater Grave." Doug Meek Photography, September 2012. Accessed August 18, 2016. www.dougmeek.com/keyword/Yoshio%20 Hosobuchi.

Mims, Bob, and Erin Alberty. "Citation Dropped against Husband of BASE Jumper in Fatal Fall." *Salt Lake Tribune*, February 13, 2014. Accessed August 21, 2016. http://archive.sltrib.com/story.php?ref=/sltrib/news/ 57534645-78/butler-park-baltrus-base.html.csp.

Mims, Bob, and Michael McFall. "Man, 74, Dies after Hanging by Foot Overnight in Zion NP Canyon." *Salt Lake Tribune*, September 21, 2012. Accessed August 18, 2016. http://archive.sltrib.com/story.php?ref=/sltrib/ news/54933651-78/canyon-hosobuchi-park-zion.html.csp.

"Peak Scaler Dies in Zion Park Plunge." *Garfield County News*, July 31, 1931. Accessed August 27, 2016. https://newspapers.lib.utah.edu/details? id=3190626&q=%22Peak+Scaler+Dies+in+Zion+Park+Plunge%22& eq=&page=1&rows=50&core=udn&fd=title_t%2Cpaper_t%2Cdate_ tdt%2Ctype_t&sort=date_tdt+asc#t_3190626.

Rizzo, Russ. "California Man Killed in Zion National Park Fall." *Salt Lake Tribune*, June 6, 2007. Accessed August 18, 2016. http://archive.sltrib .com/story.php?ref=/news/ci_6073540.

Scott, Kimberly. "Man Falls to His Death in Zion National Park." *St. George News*, July 12, 2015. Accessed August 19, 2016. www.stgeorgeutah.com/ news/archive/2015/07/12/kss-man-falls-to-his-death-in-zion-national -park.

"Sean Leary Killed in BASE Accident." *Climbing*, March 24, 2014. Accessed August 21, 2016. www.climbing.com/news/sean-leary-killed-in-base -accident.

"Skull of Cliff Dweller Found on Throne." *Iron County Record*, August 19, 1931. Accessed August 16, 2016. https://newspapers.lib.utah.edu/

details?id=3784868&q=Don+Orcutt+death&eq=&page=1&rows=50&
core=udn&fd=title_t%2Cpaper_t%2Cdate_tdt%2Ctype_t#t_3784868.

St. Germain, Patrice. "Man Dies in Rappelling Accident: Apparent Rope
Failure Causes Man to Fall in Zion Park." *Spectrum* (St. George, UT),
May 22, 2002, as posted on the Canyon Collective discussion forum.
Accessed August 17, 2016. http://canyoncollective.com/threads/zion
-fatality.3117.

"Utah Official Dies of Injuries." *Spokesman-Review*, October 13, 1992.
Accessed August 17, 2016. https://news.google.com/newspapers?nid
=1314&dat=19921013&id=G0xXAAAAIBAJ&sjid=PfADAAAAIB
AJ&pg=5706,2144338&hl=en.

Van Leuven, Chris, and Corey Buhay. "Remembering Eric Klimt." *Alpinist*,
March 21, 2016. Accessed August 20, 2016. www.alpinist.com/doc/
web16a/newswire-remembering-eric-klimt.

"What Happened in Heaps Canyon?" Discussion thread on Bogley.com, June
7, 2007. Accessed August 17, 2016. www.bogley.com/forum/showthread
.php?26059-What-happened-in-Heaps-Canyon/page4.

"Zion Climbing Fatality." SuperTopo discussion board, October 17–22, 2008.
Accessed August 18, 2016. www.supertopo.com/climbing/thread.php
?topic_id=701629&tn=40.

"Zion National Park BASE Jumper Recovered and Identified." National Park
Service news release, March 25, 2014. Accessed August 21, 2016. www
.nps.gov/zion/learn/news/basejumperrecovered.htm.

"Zion National Park (UT) Falling Fatality in Behunin Canyon." National Park
Service Morning Report, posted to Yahoo Canyons Group, located on
CanyonCollective.com, September 10, 2003. Accessed August 17, 2016.
http://canyoncollective.com/threads/more-on-the-fatality.4750/#post
-15222.

"Zion National Park Visitation 2006–2016." National Park Service. Accessed
August 18, 2016. www.nps.gov/zion/learn/management/upload/
ZION-VISITATION-2006-2016-6.pdf.

"Zion Rock Climber Falls 150 Feet to Her Death." *Deseret News*, January 23,
1999. Accessed August 17, 2016. http://beta.deseretnews.com/article/
676181/Zion-rock-climber-falls-150-feet-to-her-death.html.

Chapter 6

"2 bikers who died ID'd as S.L., Dixie residents." *Deseret News*, March 30,
2004. Accessed August 24, 2016. www.deseretnews.com/article/
595052507/2-bikers-who-died-IDd-as-SL-Dixie-residents.html.

"94-400–Zion (Utah)–MVA with Fatality." Utah Canyoneering History:
Morning Report Excerpts–1994, CanyoneeringUSA.com. Accessed
August 24, 2016. www.canyoneeringusa.com/history/mr1994.htm.

Associated Press. "Phoenix Cyclist Killed, 2 Hurt in Utah Park Tunnel." *Arizona Republic*, May 27, 1974. Accessed August 24, 2016. www.news papers.com/image/117988743.

———. "Two Motorcyclists Killed in Tunnel Crash." KSL.com, March 29, 2004. Accessed August 24, 2016. www.ksl.com/?nid=148&sid=85631.

"Death in Park Held Accident." *Deseret News*, August 28, 1958. Accessed August 23, 2016. https://news.google.com/newspapers?nid=336&dat =19580828&id=n3svAAAAIBAJ&sjid=PUgDAAAAIBAJ&pg =5014,5141538&hl=en.

"Five Die in Traffic in State; 2 Burned." *Tucson Daily Citizen*, May 27, 1974. Accessed August 23, 2016. www.newspapers.com/image/17960521/ ?terms=%22Zion%2BNational%2BPark%22%2Bdeath.

Garate, Donald T. *The Zion Tunnel: From Slickrock to Switchback*. Springdale, UT: Zion Natural History Association, 1989, pp. 19–29.

Green, Mark. "Man Seriously Injured as 8 Attempt to Illegally Bicycle Ride through Tunnel at Zion National Park." Fox 13 News, Salt Lake City, February 22, 2014. Accessed August 24, 2016. http://fox13now.com/ 2014/02/22/man-seriously-injured-as-8-attempt-to-illegally-cycle -through-tunnel-at-zion-national-park.

"Laborer Struck by Rock Dies of Hurts." *Salt Lake Telegram*, January 20, 1928. Accessed August 23, 2016. https://newspapers.lib.utah.edu/details?id =15517725&q=Mac+McClain&eq=&page=3&rows=25&core=udn& fd=title_t%2Cpaper_t%2Cdate_tdt%2Ctype_t&sort=date_tdt+asc& gallery=&date_tdt=%5B+1928-01-01T00%3A00%3A00Z+TO+1931 -12-31T00%3A00%3A00Z+%5D#t_15517725.

"Mount Carmel Tunnel Opens Scenic Beauty to Motorist." *Arizona Republic*, July 6, 1930. Accessed August 23, 2016. www.newspapers.com/image/ 116961169.

"N.M. Woman, Infant Son Killed in Canyon Crash; Injuries Claim Bicyclist." *Deseret News*, April 18, 1986. Accessed August 24, 2016. https://news .google.com/newspapers?nid=336&dat=19860418&id=K0xTAAAAIB AJ&sjid=3YMDAAAAIBAJ&pg=5217,851095&hl=en.

"Road Worker Loses Life." *Iron County Record*, January 20, 1928. Accessed August 28, 2016. https://newspapers.lib.utah.edu/details?id=3749071&q =McClain&eq=&page=1&rows=50&core=udn&fd=title_t%2Cpaper _t%2Cdate_tdt%2Ctype_t&sort=date_tdt+asc&gallery=&date_tdt= %5B+1928-01-01T00%3A00%3A00Z+TO+1928-12-31T00%3A00%3 A00Z+%5D#t_3749071.

Roy Bieghler and Joanne Hoff v. Thomas S. Kleppe, Secretary of the Interior, United States of America, and the United States of America, 633 F.2d 531 (9th Cir. 1980). Accessed on CourtListener.com, August 24, 2016. www.courtlistener.com/opinion/383572/roy-bieghler-and-joanne -hoff-v-thomas-s-kleppe-secretary-of-the/?stat_Non-Precedential

=on&sort=score+desc&stat_Relating-to+orders=on&court_cadc=on&stat
_Precedential=on&stat_Errata=on&page=101.

United Press International. "Tunnel Design Caused Motorcycle Crashes,
Attorney Says in Suit." *Arizona Republic*, April 15, 1982. Accessed
August 24, 2016. www.newspapers.com/image/121496678.

———. "Utahn, Californian Die in Motorcycle Mishaps." *Ogden Standard-
Examiner*, June 7, 1972. Accessed August 23, 2016. www.newspapers
.com/image/31537133.

"Zion–Mt. Carmel Highway and Tunnel." Zion National Park website.
Accessed August 23, 2016. www.nps.gov/zion/learn/historyculture/
zmchighway.htm.

"Zion National Park (UT) Two Motorcyclists Killed in Tunnel." Zion Morning Report, March 31, 2004, located on CanyonCollective.com. Accessed
August 24, 2016. http://canyoncollective.com/threads/zion-morning
-report.5197.

CHAPTER 7

Anastasia, George. "Suit Targets Man Acquitted in Wife's Death." Philly.com,
September 18, 2003. Accessed August 25, 2016. http://articles.philly
.com/2003-09-18/news/25457997_1_civil-action-civil-complaint-death.

Associated Press. "Defense Expert Gives Harmful Testimony in Zion Death
Trial." *Daily Herald*, November 21, 2002. Accessed August 25, 2016.
www.heraldextra.com/news/local/defense-expert-gives-harmful
-testimony-in-zion-death-trial/article_3af9a2d2-b7a7-5a53-bdbb
-629f17087157.html.

———. "Trial Begins for Hiker Accused of Pushing Wife to Death." *Kingman
Daily Miner*, November 7, 2002. Accessed August 25, 2016. https://news
.google.com/newspapers?nid=932&dat=20021107&id=wscvAAAAIB
AJ&sjid=O1MDAAAAIBAJ&pg=3706,4391642&hl=en.

Braun, Joe. "Observation Point Trail." Joe's Guide to Zion National Park.
Accessed August 28, 2016. www.citrusmilo.com/zionguide/obspoint.cfm.

Dobner, Jennifer. "Sister Had Questions over Hiker's Death in Fall." *Deseret
News*, November 19, 2002. Accessed August 24, 2016. https://news
.google.com/newspapers?nid=336&dat=20021119&id=nB5OAAAA
IBAJ&sjid=G-0DAAAAIBAJ&pg=6787,2234565&hl=en.

———. "Statements Don't Add Up, Ranger Says." *Deseret News*, November
20, 2002. Accessed August 25, 2016. https://news.google.com/
newspapers?nid=336&dat=20021120&id=nR5OAAAAIBAJ&sjid
=G-0DAAAAIBAJ&pg=3067,2615754&hl=en.

Lamb, William. "Camper's Death Is Under Investigation." *St. Louis Post-
Dispatch*, March 23, 2004. Accessed August 25, 2016. www.newspapers
.com/image/151791851.

Saidi, Nicole. "Utah Police Investigate Student's Death." ASU Web Devil, April 1, 2004. Accessed August 25, 2016. https://asuwebdevilarchive.asu .edu/issues/2004/04/01/news/647652.

Soto, Onell R. "Former S.D. Man Acquitted in Wife's Fatal Fall off Cliff." San Diego Union-Tribune, November 27, 2002. Accessed August 25, 2016. http://legacy.sandiegouniontribune.com/news/metro/20021127-9999 _2m27cliff.html.

"Sued in Wife's Death." Reading Eagle, February 15, 2003. Accessed August 24, 2016. https://news.google.com/newspapers?nid=1955&dat=20030215 &id=WPohAAAAIBAJ&sjid=SaMFAAAAIBAJ&pg=3402,8304037 &hl=en.

TOBO Investment Partnership vs. Bottarini, GIN027607. Superior Court of California, County of San Diego, North County Judicial Branch. February 10, 2003.

Welling, Angie. "2 Jurors Persuaded Others to Acquit Bottarini." Deseret News, November 27, 2002. Accessed August 25, 2016. https://news.google .com/newspapers?nid=336&dat=20021127&id=oh5OAAAAIBAJ& sjid=G-0DAAAAIBAJ&pg=6738,6508395&hl=en.

———. "Blood Spot on Cliff Presented at Trial." Deseret News, November 8, 2002. Accessed August 25, 2016. https://news.google.com/newspapers ?nid=336&dat=20021108&id=lh5OAAAAIBAJ&sjid=_-wDAAAAI BAJ&pg=6982,3971689&hl=en.

———. "Bottarini Denies Pushing Wife off Cliff." Deseret News, November 23, 2002. Accessed August 25, 2016. http://beta.deseretnews.com/article/ 950157/Bottarini-denies-pushing-wife-off-cliff.html?pg=all.

———. "Bottarini Is Cleared of All Charges." Deseret News, November 26, 2002. Accessed August 25, 2016. https://news.google.com/newspapers ?id=oR5OAAAAIBAJ&sjid=G-0DAAAAIBAJ&pg=2462%2C6006488.

———. "Death Hit Bottarini Hard, Kin Say." Deseret News, November 22, 2002. Accessed August 25, 2016. https://news.google.com/newspapers ?nid=336&dat=20021122&id=nx5OAAAAIBAJ&sjid=G-0DAAAAI BAJ&pg=2124,3471790&hl=en.

———. "Hiker Tells of Finding Body on Trail." Deseret News, November 7, 2002. Accessed August 24, 2016. http://beta.deseretnews.com/article/ 947325/Hiker-tells-of-finding-body-on-trail.html.

———. "Juror Cites Miscue in Bottarini Acquittal." Deseret News, December 4, 2002. Accessed August 25, 2016. http://beta.deseretnews.com/article/ 952076/Juror-cites-miscue-in-Bottarini-acquittal.html.

———. "Jury Told to Put Itself in Bottarini's Shoes." Deseret News, November 25, 2002. Accessed August 25, 2016. http://beta.deseretnews.com/ article/950584/Jury-told-to-put-itself-in-Bottarinis-shoes.html.

———. "Trial Begins in Hiking Death." Deseret News, November 5, 2002. Accessed August 25, 2016. https://news.google.com/newspapers

?nid=336&dat=20021105&id=lB5OAAAAIBAJ&sjid=_-wDAAAAI
BAJ&pg=3151,2702405&hl=en.

CHAPTER 8

"Bergemeyer, Frederick R., 1913–1952." Obituary, *Mason City Globe Gazette*,
August 29, 1952, as reposted at IAGenWeb.org. Accessed August 25,
2016. http://iagenweb.org/boards/floyd/obituaries/index.cgi?read
=396804.

Charnock, Richard. "3 Bodies, Wreckage of Plane Found in Utah Canyon."
Arizona Republic, November 10, 1987. Accessed August 25, 2016. www
.newspapers.com/image/121136802/?terms=%22Zion%2BNational%2
BPark%22%2Bdeath.

"Clair Hirschi Buried at Rockville on Monday, August 23." *Washington County
News*, August 26, 1937. Accessed August 25, 2016. https://newspapers
.lib.utah.edu/details?id=21821961&q=Clair+Hirschi+death+August+23
+1937&eq=&page=1&rows=25&core=udn&fd=title_t%2Cpaper_t%2
Cdate_tdt%2Ctype_t&sort=rel&gallery=&date_tdt=%5B+1937-01
-01T00%3A00%3A00Z+TO+1937-12-31T00%3A00%3A00Z+%5
D&facet_type=death#t_21821961.

"Echo Accident Kills Woman; 3 Others Dead." *Ogden Standard-Examiner*,
August 24, 1952. Accessed August 25, 2016. www.newspapers.com/
image/?spot=5958855.

McAuliffe, Bill. "Minnesota Model T Enthusiast Killed in Crash of Antique
Car." *Minneapolis Star Tribune*, July 26, 2013. Accessed August 25, 2016.
www.startribune.com/minnesota-model-t-enthusiast-killed-in-crash-of
-antique-car/217193941.

"N9447B Accident Description." PlaneCrashMap.com. Accessed August 25,
2016. http://planecrashmap.com/plane/ut/N9447B.

"NTSB Identification: DEN88FA023." Aviation Accidents in Washington
County, Washington County Historical Society. Accessed August 25,
2016. http://wchsutah.org/aviation/aviation-accidents-1987-11-06.txt.

Reavy, Pat. "1 Killed, 3 Injured in Model T Crash Near Zion National Park."
Deseret News, July 26, 2013. Accessed August 25, 2016. http://beta
.deseretnews.com/article/865583682/Antique-car-crashes-near-Zion-4
-injured.html.

Rindels, Michelle. "Model T Overturns, Kills 1." *Decatur Herald and Review*,
July 27, 2013. Accessed August 25, 2016. www.newspapers.com/image/
84393378/?terms=%22Zion%2BNational%2BPark%22%2Bdeath.

United Press International. "Two Die in Zion Rollover." *Daily Herald* (Provo,
UT), July 24, 1967. Accessed August 25, 2016. www.newspapers.com/
image/25598848/?terms=Columbus%2BOhio%2BThomas%2BNewman.

"Utah Mishaps Take 2 Lives." *Salt Lake Telegram*, August 23, 1937.
Accessed August 25, 2016. https://newspapers.lib.utah.edu/

details?id=18683883&q=Clair+Hirschi+death&eq=&page=1&rows=50&
core=udn&fd=title_t%2Cpaper_t%2Cdate_tdt%2Ctype_t&sort=&
gallery=&date_tdt=%5B+1930-01-01T00%3A00%3A00Z+TO+1941
-12-31T00%3A00%3A00Z+%5D#t_18683883.

"Zion's Ranger Killed on Trail in Park." *Salt Lake Tribune*, August 24, 1952.
Accessed August 25, 2016. www.newspapers.com/image/12896949.

CHAPTER 9

"Body Found Beneath Canyon Overlook in Zion National Park." National
Park Service news release, February 26, 2009. Accessed August 27, 2016.
www.nps.gov/zion/learn/news/body-found-beneath-canyon-overlook-in
-zion-national-park.htm.

"Civilian Conservation Corps." Zion National Park website. Accessed August
26, 2016. www.nps.gov/zion/learn/historyculture/civilian-conservation
-corps.htm.

"Death Stalks Picnic Party at Zion Park." *Washington County News*, April 17,
1930. Accessed August 26, 2016. https://newspapers.lib.utah.edu/
details?id=21779738&q=Albin+Brooksby&eq=&page=1&rows
=50&core=udn&fd=title_t%2Cpaper_t%2Cdate_tdt%2Ctype_t&sort
=&gallery=&date_tdt=%5B+1929-01-01T00%3A00%3A00Z+TO+1931
-12-31T00%3A00%3A00Z+%5D&facet_paper=Washington+County+
News#t_21779738.

"Falling Fatality Victim at Zion National Park Identified." National Park
Service news release, February 27, 2009. Accessed August 27, 2016.
www.nps.gov/zion/learn/news/falling-fatality-victim-at-zion-national
-park-identified.htm.

"FBI Identifies Dead Woman Found in National Park." *Nevada State Journal*, July 12, 1947. Accessed August 27, 2016. www.newspapers.com/
image/75094140/?terms=Evelyn%2BCallahan%2Bdeath%2BZion.

"FBI Identifies Victim of Zion Park Slaying." *Salt Lake Telegram*, July 11,
1947. Accessed August 27, 2016. https://newspapers.lib.utah.edu/
details?id=17330199&q=death+Zion+Park&eq=&page=1&rows=50&
core=udn&fd=title_t%2Cpaper_t%2Cdate_tdt%2Ctype_t&sort=&
gallery=#t_17330199.

"Friends and Family Remember Corey Buxton." Las Vegas Now (CBS Chan-
nel 8), July 25, 2010. Accessed August 28, 2016. www.lasvegasnow.com/
news/friends-and-family-remember-corey-buxton.

"Hero Loses Life in Fire on Zion Mount'n." *Washington County News*, December 22, 1921. Accessed August 26, 2016. https://newspapers.lib.utah.edu/
details?id=21922891&q=Ether+Winder&eq=&page=2&rows=25&core
=udn&fd=title_t%2Cpaper_t%2Cdate_tdt%2Ctype_t&sort=date_tdt+
asc&gallery=&date_tdt=%5B+1921-01-01T00%3A00%3A00Z+TO+

1923-12-31T00%3A00%3A00Z+%5D&facet_paper=Washington
+County+News#t_21922891.

"Historic Cable Mountain Draw Works Stabilization Project Completed."
National Park Service news release, January 13, 2011. Accessed August
26, 2016. www.nps.gov/zion/learn/news/historic-cable-mountain
-draw-works-stabilization-project-completed.htm.

"Hop Valley Trail." Zion National Park website. Accessed August 27, 2016.
www.nps.gov/zion/planyourvisit/hop-valley-trail.htm.

"Leg Injury Proves Fatal to CCC Enrollee." *Washington County News*, February
17, 1938. Accessed August 26, 2016. https://newspapers.lib.utah.edu/
details?id=21810187&q=Leg+Injury+Proves+Fatal+to+CCC+Enrollee
&eq=&page=10&rows=50&core=udn&fd=title_t%2Cpaper_t%2Cdate_
tdt%2Ctype_t&sort=date_tdt+asc&gallery=&date_tdt=%5B+1938-01
-01T00%3A00%3A00Z+TO+1938-12-31T00%3A00%3A00Z+%5D
&facet_paper=Washington+County+News#t_21810187.

Lemmon, D. W., Enos E. Winder, Eliel Winder, and John A. Allred. "Further
Particulars of Ether Winder's Death." *Washington County News*, January
12, 1922. Accessed August 26, 2016. https://newspapers.lib.utah.edu/
details?id=21925343&q=Ether+Winder&eq=&page=2&rows=25&core
=udn&fd=title_t%2Cpaper_t%2Cdate_tdt%2Ctype_t&sort=date_tdt+
asc&gallery=&date_tdt=%5B+1921-01-01T00%3A00%3A00Z+TO+
1923-12-31T00%3A00%3A00Z+%5D&facet_paper=Washington+
County+News#t_21925343.

"Oregon Woman Slain by Bullet." *News-Review* (Roseburg, OR), July 12,
1947. Accessed August 27, 2016. www.newspapers.com/image/
96963405/?terms=%22Zion%2BNational%2BPark%22%2Bdeath.

"Particulars of Winder's Death on Zion Mountain." *Washington County News*,
December 29, 1921. Accessed August 26, 2016. https://newspapers.lib
.utah.edu/details?id=21923398&q=Ether+Winder&eq=&page=2&rows
=25&core=udn&fd=title_t%2Cpaper_t%2Cdate_tdt%2Ctype_t&sort=
date_tdt+asc&gallery=&date_tdt=%5B+1921-01-01T00%3A00%3
A00Z+TO+1923-12-31T00%3A00%3A00Z+%5D&facet_paper
=Washington+County+News#t_21923398.

"Suicide Angel Advanced in Zion Death." *Salt Lake Telegram*, July 16,
1947. Accessed August 27, 2016. https://newspapers.lib.utah.edu/
details?id=17331193&q=death+Zion+Park&eq=&page=1&rows=50&
core=udn&fd=title_t%2Cpaper_t%2Cdate_tdt%2Ctype_t&sort=&
gallery=#t_17331193.

Taylor, Tiffany. Zion National Park. Charleston, SC: Arcadia, 2008. Pages
58–60 accessed through Google Books, August 26, 2016. https://books
.google.com/books?id=S6FPDKFnzE4C&pg=PA60&lpg=PA60&dq
=Thornton+Hepworth+1908&source=bl&ots=5zJ_8XYvLa&sig=Tp4gaN
_cv6mgf7bnMre0dDqMs60&hl=en&sa=X&ved=0ahUKEwiC4IH0r4

XOAhVLaz4KHSBeAl0Q6AEINDAF#v=onepage&q=Thornton%20
Hepworth%201908&f=false.

Vartabedian, Ralph. "For Boy Scouts, Trails Can Lead to Danger." *Los Angeles Times*, December 5, 2010. Accessed August 27, 2016. http://articles .latimes.com/2010/dec/05/nation/la-na-scouts-20101205/2.

"Woman Slain in Zion Park Is Identified." *Deseret News*, July 11, 1947. Accessed August 27, 2016. https://news.google.com/newspapers?nid =336&dat=19470711&id=vNdSAAAAIBAJ&sjid=zX8DAAAAIBA J&pg=3376,1072628&hl=en.

INDEX

ability overestimation, 104–8
Adams, Jake, 101
Adams, Karen, 40
Aeolus (Greek mythological location), 48
air plane crashes, 148–50
Aldisert, Ruggero J., 89
Algan, Ramsey E., 6
Anderson, Albert, 15
Anderson, Kaden, 44
Anderson, Steve, 93
Andrew, Bob, 52
Angels Landing (*formerly known as*
    Temple of Aeolus)
  descriptions, 48
  falls off trails to, 55–56, 61–63, 63–64,
    64–65, 66–67
  falls over cliffs at, 58–61
  falls over viewpoint cliffs to, 57–58,
    67–68
  heart attacks on, 56–57
  name history, 48–49
  popularity of, 61
  rappelling accidents, 53–55
  safety precautions and warnings, 68
  safety restriction debates, 64
  suicides on, 57–58, 161
  suspicious deaths on, 51–53
  trails to, 49–50
Angels Landing Trail (the neck/the
    chains), 49–50, 61–63, 63–64,
    64–65, 66–67
animals
  dogs for search and rescue, 6, 16, 44,
    162
  horses for search and rescue, 150
  wildlife safety guidelines, 172–74
Arthur, Linda, 38, 44
Arthur, Steve, 38, 43
Artmann, Bryan, 110–11
ascenders, mechanical, 102–3

automobiles, 165, 173. *See also* vehicular
    accidents

backcountry
  falls over cliffs at night, 77–78
  permits issued to, statistics, 39
  safety precautions, 164, 165–68
  solo, 79–80
Baltrus, Aly, 106, 107
Banach, Mike, 107
bandanas, 169
Bangerter, John, 15
Barlow, David, 118
Barlow, Guy, 128
Barnes, Dick, 13
barriers, 71, 165
BASE (Building, Antenna, Span, Earth)
    jumping
  deaths due to, 116–17, 119–20
  prohibitions on, 117–18, 120
  sport descriptions, 116, 120
Baty, Bonnie, 85
Beehives, 46
Behunin Canyon, 95–96, 109
Bellows, Amber, 116–18
Bergemeyer, Fred E., 145–46
bets, 58–61
Bevins, Phil, 163
bicycle riders, 128, 130–31, 165
Biedermann, Keith, 101–2
Bieghler, Roy W., 126–28
Bonanno, Tony, 77, 78
Bottarini, James
  charges and trial, 138–41
  civil suits and countersuits, 141–42
  gambling, 139
  hike and accident accounts, 132–33,
    136–37
  marriage issues, 132
  post-accident behavior, 134–37

wife's insurance policy and family trust, 137, 138
Bottarini, Patricia
  death and investigation, 132–37
  marriage issues, 132
  trial and civil suits, 138–42
Bourne, David, 77–78
Boutillet, Everett, 112–13
Boyack, Al, 51
Boy Scouts, 58–61, 162–63
Braun, Joe, 2, 132–33
Brereton, Thomas, 78
Brewer, Mark, 24, 27–32
Brigham, David, 161
Brooksby, Albin, 93, 156–57
Browning, Robert, 73–74
Brueck, Fred, 74
Brum, Robin, 38, 39, 44
Bryant, David Faulkner, 93–94
Bryce Canyon National Park, 123
Buccello, David, 6, 33, 54, 55
Buccello, Pat, 136, 137
Buhay, Corey, 114, 115
Butler, Clayton, 116–18, 121
Buxton, Corey, 162–63

Cable Mountain
  cable system detachment, 156–57
  fires, 153–56
  lightning, 152–53
  lumber industry history and cable works, 152
cable works, 151–53, 156–57
Cafferata, Christine, 69
Cafferata, Eugene, 69–71
Callahan, Ann Theresa, 161
Callahan, Evelyn Frances, 159–61
Callahan, Hugh M., 161
Campbell, Glen, 149
camping, 77–78, 165
canyoneering
  accident causes, common, 100–101
  canyon descriptions, 1–2, 24–25
  ethical practices for, 39
  experience requirements, 104, 107–8
  fall due to lost balance, 95
  flash flood dangers, overview, 4, 8
  flash flood tragedies at Keyhole Canyon, 38–45

flash flood tragedies at Narrows on Virgin River, 10–17, 18–21, 21–23
flash flood tragedies on Kolob Creek, 24–37
gear recommendations, 2
history of, 94–95
permit requirements, 165–66
rappelling accidents, 95–96, 96–100, 101–2, 105–8
water safety guidelines, 170–72
Canyon Overlook Trail, 46–47, 161–62
Carpenter, Hayden, 114
Carroll, Henry, 157
Casalou, Robert, 76
Caseiro, Marie, 80
Cassell, B. J., 38
Cathedral Mountain, 92–93
CFS (cubic feet per second), 19–20, 42
chains, as trail guides, 49–50, 68, 70, 83, 88
Chicken-Out Point, 49. See also Scout Lookout
Chidester, Daniel, 18–21, 68
children. See also teenagers
  falls off trails over cliffs, 75–76
  falls off waterfall ledges, 76
  lightning deaths, 153
  safety guidelines with, 46, 72, 173
  slickrock streams and falls over waterfalls, 86–88
  trail flooding over cliffs, 45–47
Childs, Doug, 14, 15
Chin, Norman, 77
Christensen, John Michael, 53–55
Church of Jesus Christ of Latter-day Saints (Mormons)
  Boy Scout hikers, 59
  cable system victims, 157
  Explorer Scouts and flash flood tragedy, 24, 26–32, 36
  lawsuits against, 61
  lawsuits and beliefs, 34
  rappelling accident victims, 55
Civilian Conservation Corps, 157–59
Clark, I. F., 158
Classic Helicopter, 112
Clear Creek, 38, 41–42, 43
Clery, Jim, 41–42
Climbing (magazine), 119

climbing and climbing accidents
   on Angels Landing, 53–55
   causes, overview, 100–101
   falls, 93, 108, 109–10, 110–11
   first park death, 92–93
   permit requirements, 165
   technical issues, 93–94, 96–103,
      113–15
clothing, 2, 167, 171
Collard, Kathryn, 88
Collins, Lynn, 35
compasses, 167
Connors, Richard, 96–100
construction accidents, 124–25, 158–59
Cook Charles, 37
Cooke, James F., 128
cotton clothing, 171
Cottrell, Lane Kelton, 72–73
Court of the Patriarchs, 78
Cox, Donald, 133–34
Cox, Glenda, 133–34
creeks. *See also specific names of creeks*
   descriptions, 24–26, 38
   flash flood tragedies, 11, 24, 26–37
   rainstorms and flooding of, 46
   water safety guidelines for, 170–72
cubic feet per second (CFS), 19–20, 42

Dahl, Laura, 38
dams, 33, 35–37
Darger, Bonnie, 15
Davies, Denny, 6–7, 87
Davis, Kevin, 130
Dearden, Allen, 15
Dearden, John, 10, 15
Deep Creek, 18
Deep Creek Wilderness Study, 25
Deer Trap Mountain, 73
DeMasters, Tiffany, 57
Denali Nation Park, 36–37, 79, 91
desert conditions, 45–46, 169–70
disorientation, 170
DNA testing, 17
dogs, 6, 16, 44, 162
Doria, Rene, 59
Dougan, David H., III, 141
Draw Works cable system, 151–53,
      156–57
driving, 165, 173

drowning, 5–7, 10–17, 24–32, 38–45
Dwyer, Jeffrey Robert, 51–53
Dyer, Marco, 129–30
dynamite blasts, 158–59
dynamite fumes, 125

Eaker, David, 23, 43
East Rim Trail, 77
East Temple, 46
Eggertz, Brittany, 86–87
Eggertz, Jeffrey, 86, 87–88
Eggertz, Lora, 87
Eggertz, Tyler Jeffrey, 86–88
Elder, Nancy, 88
Ellis, Kim, 26–27, 32
Ellis, Shane, 26, 28
Emerald Pools, 69–71, 76, 78, 86–88,
      159–60
Employee Falls, 79
employees, park, 72, 73, 79
EMS (emergency medical service), 110,
      111
Engibous, Mark, 108
equipment. *See* gear
Ertischek, Mark, 56–57
Explorer Scouts, 24, 26–32, 36
*Exploring the Backcountry of Zion National
   Park* (Brereton), 78

Falk, Robert, 134–35, 136
Falling Water Hanging Gardens Cliffs, 95
Farley, Mike, 63
fatigue, 102
Faust, John, 69
Faust, Rose, 69
Favela, Gary, 38, 44
Federal Bureau of Investigation (FBI),
      52–53, 159, 160
Felling, Christopher, 64
Felton, James, 75
fences, 71, 165
Fieden, Lila, 15
fig-eight knots, 99–100
fires, 153–56
firestarters, 167
first-aid supplies, 167
Fisher, Frederick Vining, 48–49
Flanigan, David, 151–52
flashlights, 167

Fleischer, Dave, 26, 27–30, 32
floods, flash. *See also* Kolob Creek flash
    flood
  descriptions, 4
  Keyhole Canyon, 38–45
  Narrows/Virgin River, 5–6, 8, 10–17,
    18–21, 21–23
  park policies and safety, 37, 45
  safety guidelines for, 170–72
  safety information and warnings, 7–9,
    37, 170
  signs indicating, 170–71
  trail dangers and cliff falls, 45–47
Florence, Steve, 14, 15
food and snacks, 167, 169, 171, 172
Forster, Craig, 84–86
Frankewicz, Christopher, 95–96
freak accidents, 95, 125
Freebairn, Doralee, 17
Fulton, Mike, 134
Furstnow, Russ, 148

Garcia, Paul, 7
gear
  for canyoneering, 2
  climbing and technical issues with,
    93–94, 96–103, 113–15
  food and snacks, 167, 169, 171, 172
  for hiking, 166–68, 169, 171
  permit requirements, 18, 35–36
  for spring weather, 80
  water and water treatment tools,
    167–68, 169, 171
ghosting, 39
Gifford, Gerald, 76
Glacier National Park, 80
Goebel, John, 142–43
Goldstein, Barry S., 63–64
Grand Canyon National Park, 109, 117,
  120, 123
Great Arch, 161
Great White Throne, 49, 72–73, 90–92,
  91
Grim, Katherine, 15
Grunig, Michael, 66
Grunig, Rick, 66
Grunig, Tammy, 66–67
guardrails, 71, 165
guns, 160

Haas, Cheri, 109
Half Dome (Yosemite National Park), 37
Haraden, Tom, 56, 57
Harmon, Carol, 15
Harris, Lynn, 61
Harrison, Dana, 75–76
Harrison, Max, 75
Harrison, Richard, 75
Harrison, Rick, 118–19
hats, 169
Hawkes, Jalaine, 147
headlamps, 167
Heaps Canyon, 101–2, 110–11
heart attacks, 56–57
heat exhaustion, 169–70
heat stroke, 162–63, 170
helicopters, 81, 94, 109, 112, 117, 120
helmets, 109, 110
Hepworth, Thornton, Jr., 153
Hidden Canyon, 83–84
hiking. *See also* canyoneering
  falls over cliffs at night, 69–71, 78
  falls over cliffs at viewpoint, 57–58,
    67–68
  falls over cliffs due to lost footing, 78,
    84–86
  falls over cliffs due to peer pressure,
    58–61
  falls over cliffs due to trail flooding
    slides, 45–47
  falls over cliffs from ice slips, 80–81
  falls over cliffs off Angels Landing
    neck trail, 61–63, 63–64, 64–65,
    66–67
  falls over cliffs wandering off-trail,
    55–56, 72–73, 109
  falls over cliffs while photographing,
    77
  gear recommendations, 2, 166–67
  heart attacks while, 56–57
  hyperthermia, 162–63
  safety guidelines for, 164, 165–68,
    169–70
  slickrock falls over cliffs, 83–84, 109
  slickrock falls over waterfalls, 76,
    86–88
  solo, 79–83, 165, 173
  suspicious deaths while, 51–53, 132–42
  trail dangers, overview, 72

trail descriptions, 48–51, 132–33
Hillery, Allen R., 93
Hillery, Ronald, 93
Hilton, Kelly, 73–74
Hinton, Rymal, 81
Hippotes (Greek mythological figure), 48
Hirschi, Arden, 145
Hirschi, Clair L., 144–45
Hirschi, Claud, 49
Hirschi, Heber, 145
Hoff, Harvey Frank, 126–28
Hoff, Joanne, 126–28
Holley, Joseph, 71
Hooker, Robert, 102
Hop Valley, 162–63
horses, 150
Hosobuchi, Dresden, 105–8
Hosobuchi, Yoshio, 105–8
Howard-Jones, Carolyn, 132, 136–37,
    137–38
Humphries, Glenwood, 6, 52
Hurd, Lyle David, III, 108
hydration, 169
Hyland, Dallas, 112–13
hyperthermia (heat stroke), 162–63, 170
hypothermia, 2, 9, 22, 171–72

Imlay Canyon, 111–13
Iverson, Jimmy, 73–74

Jensen, Frank, 74
Joe's Guide to Zion National Park
    (website), 2, 132–33
Johnson, Christian Louis, 112–13
Johnson, Frank, 14, 15–17
Johnson, Karen, 147–48
Johnson, Tim, 147–48
Jones, Kristoffer, 58–61
Jones, Ruth, 61
Jones, Tom, 25–26, 50, 101
judgment and common sense, 9
jumars (mechanical ascenders), 102–3
Justett, Vance, 13

Kaiser, Dorothy, 57–58, 161
Katwok, Thomas, 15
Katz, Paul A., 127
Keller, Michelle, 149
Keyhole Canyon, 38–45

Klimt, Carl, 115
Klimt, Eric Michael, 113–15
knives, 167
knots, fig-eight, 99–100
Kolob Canyon, 80, 148–50
Kolob Creek flash flood (1993)
    flash flood cause, 33
    flash flood tragedies at, 24, 26–32
    hiking route and area descriptions,
        24–26
    information center at, 25
    lawsuits, 33–37
    search and recovery, 32–33
Kolob Reservoir dam, 33
Kolob Technical Canyons, 24–25
Kuhlmann, Peter, 137

Lady Mountain, 70–71, 75–76
Lambert, Richard, 139
Langston, Clarinda, 153
LaPlante, Matthew D., 60
Largay, Geraldine, 80
Larson, Carla, 11, 15
Larson, Rich, 26
La Verkin Creek, 25
lawsuits, 33–37, 61, 88–89, 126–28
Leary, Sean, 119–20
Lemmon, Clarence, 153–56
Lewis, Penny, 82
lightning, 37, 152–53
Lodge Canyon, 93
Long, Mr.s Milo D., 125
Lopez, Eddie, 7
Loso, Andy, 147, 148
lumber industry and equipment, 151–53,
    156–57

MacKenzie, Mark, 39, 40, 44
Maltez, Nancy, 64–65
maps, 167
Martin, Brad, 126
matches, 167
Mather, Stephen, 123
McCafferty, Mary (Evelyn Francis
    Callahan), 159–61
McClain, Allan T., 124
McFall, Michael, 106
McGinn, Brett, 136
McIntyre, E. Clark, 144

McIntyre, Linda, 15
McIntyre, Margaret, 15
Merriman, Thad, 15
Middle Emerald Pool, 78, 86–88
Milestone, Jim, 118, 120
Miller, Steven Lee, 77
Milligan, Tanya, 46, 70
Milobedzki, Regine, 67–68
Mims, Bob, 106
mirrors, 167
Model T Ford Club, 147–48
Moonlight Buttress, 113–15
Mormons. *See* Church of Jesus Christ of
    Latter-day Saints
Morrison, Johnny, 124–25
Morrow, Colin Robert, 130
Moss, Lyle, 12, 13, 15
motorcyclists, 126–28, 129–30, 144–45
mountain lions, 173–74
Mountain of the Sun, 72–73
Mount Kinesava, 116–18
Mt. McKinley, 37
Muñoz, Michael, 45–47

Narrows of the Virgin River
    closure policies, 19
    descriptions, 1–3
    flash flood descriptions, 4
    flash flood tragedies, 4, 5–7, 8, 10–17,
        18–21, 21–23
    hiking information for, 9
    safety guidelines for, 170
    safety information and warnings, 7–9
National Park Service. *See also* permits;
    safety guidelines; search and
    recovery/rescue missions
    BASE jumping bans, 118
    death investigations, 6–7, 23, 54, 59,
        103, 136, 161–62
    tunnel planning, 123
    tunnel usage regulations, 129
    wrongful death lawsuits against, 35–37
National Register of Historic Places, 157
National Weather Service, 9, 39, 40, 170
Natural Bridge Canyon, 73–74
Nay, Josh, 26
Nelson, Alvin, 14, 15–17
Nevada Contracting Company, 123
Newman, Jean Helen, 146

Newman, John William, 146
Newman, Thomas, 146
Nichols, Ray, 14
night (darkness)
    BASE jumping at, 118–19
    camping and falls off cliffs, 77–78
    climbing during, 102
    hiking and falls off cliffs, 69–71, 78
"no rescue" zones, 36
North Creek Left Fork. *See* Subway
Northeast Buttress, 108
Not Imlay Canyon, 112
Nunes, Roberta, 119, 120

Observation Point, 132–36
Odysseus (Greek mythological figure), 48
off-trail hiking, 55–56, 72–73, 109
Orcutt, Don, 90–93
Orderville Canyon, 11–13
Outside (magazine), 27, 33, 37, 39, 44

Padilla, Aaron J., 130
Perkins, Mike, 26
permits
    danger ratings and issuance of, 35–36
    flash flood warnings, 7–8, 33–34, 35,
        39–40
    lack of, 18, 20
    requirements for, 18, 35–36, 165–66
Perry, Robert, 11–12, 15
Peterson, Robert, 76
Phillips, Affin William, 80–81
photography, 77, 172–73
Piacitelli, India, 44
Piacitelli, Jay, 44
picnics, 156–57
Pine Creek Canyon, 46, 123
plane crashes, 148–50
port-a-ledges, 102
post-traumatic stress syndrome, 34
preparation requirements, 18, 47
Price, Larry, 78
Prodigal Sun, 53–55
Profitt, Clark, 109
public works projects, 157–59
Purcell, Cindy, 39–40

rafting, 18–19, 68
railings, 71

rainstorms, 11–12, 39–40, 45–47, 148–50. *See also* floods, flash
Randall, Dave, 13
rangers
  flash flood knowledge and lawsuit, 33–34, 35
  flash flood warnings, 7–8, 21, 40
  safety guidelines and listening to, 166
rappelling accidents
  at Angels Landing, 53–55
  at Behunin Canyon, 95–96
  at Heaps Canyon, 101–2
  at Imlay Canyon, 111–13
  at Spaceshot, 96–100
  at Subway, 93–94, 105–8
  at Touchstone, 102–3
Refrigerator Canyon, 49
Reimherr, Patrick, 85
Renouf, Ray, 16–17
Renouf, Roy A., 125
reservoirs, 33, 35–37
residential history, 151
Reynolds, Muku, 38, 43–44
rivers and streams, 86–88, 170–72. *See also* Narrows of the Virgin River
Riverside Walk, 2
roads and highways, 25, 165, 173. *See also* vehicular accidents
Robertson, Von H., 158
Rock and Ice (magazine), 113
rocks, falling, 124
Rocky Mountain Rescue Dogs, 6
Romberg, Joseph, 146
Rose, Steven Michael, 126
Rowlands, Lawrence, 78
Ruesch, Walter, 49
Russell, Eugene, 157
Russell, John, 78
Rydatch, Melodyie, 118

safety guidelines and precautions
  barriers, 71–72, 88, 165
  for driving, 165
  for flash floods, 170–72
  for hiking, 164, 165–68, 169–70
  park policies and tunnel usage restrictions, 129
  park warning signs, 68, 86, 88

visitor responsibilities, 36–37, 50, 71–72, 89, 109, 168
weather warnings, 7–9, 33–34, 35, 37, 39–40, 45
salty snacks, 169
sandstone, 78, 168. *See also* slickrock conditions
satellite emergency notification devices (SENDs), 111–12
Scaffidi, Jesse, 18–21, 68
Schaffer, Grayson, 39, 44, 45
Schena, Scott, 79
Scott, Adene, 15
Scott, Walter, 13–14
Scout Lookout (Chicken-Out Point), 49, 57–58, 67–68
search and recovery/rescue missions
  airplane crashes, 150
  canyon challenges, 81
  cliff falls while hiking, 62
  costs, 37
  for flash flood victims, 6–7, 15–17, 19–20, 23, 32–33, 43–44
  with helicopters, 81, 94, 109, 112, 117, 120
  for missing hikers, 71
  of remains, 80–81
  statistics, 45
Sender, Georg, 55–56
SENDs (satellite emergency notification devices), 111–12
Sheer, Julie, 50
Simpson, Sasha, 95
skills requirements
  for hiking, 47
  knowledge of, as safety guideline, 168
  park policies and assessments of, 45
slickrock conditions
  descriptions, 73
  falls off cliffs due to, 45–47, 73–74, 83–84, 109
  lawsuits challenging safety warnings, 88–89
  river rocks, 2, 9
  safety guidelines for, 168, 172
  in streams over waterfalls, 86–88
Smith, Gaylun, 61
Smith, Kirk, 83, 96
Smith, Robert, 150

SOCOTWA Expeditions, 10–17
solo hiking
    advantages of, 79–80
    falls off cliffs while, 80–81
    group separation and falls over cliffs,
        82–83
    safety guidelines and, 165, 173
Spaceshot, 96–100
speeding, 130
Spencer, Christopher, 109–10
Spencer, Thomas, 15
Spondeck, Leif, 15
Stevens, Chris, 26
Stevens, Lee, 157
storms
    airplane crashes during, 148–50
    flash floods, 11–12, 39–42
    lightning, 37, 152–53
    safety guidelines and, 170
    trail dangers, 45–47
Stout, Lionel, 153
Streaked Wall, 46
Subway (or Left Fork of North Creek)
    climbing accidents, 93–94, 109
    inexperienced canyoneers, 105–7
    route descriptions, 38–39, 104, 107–8
    solo hiking fall off trail over cliffs,
        82–83
suicides, 57–58, 159–62
sun protection, 167, 169
suspicious deaths, 51–53, 142–43. See also
    Bottarini, James; Bottarini, Patricia
Switchbacks, 46

Tamin, Roselan "Ross," 96–100
Tanner, Ray, 158–59
Taylor Creek, South Fork of, 80–81
teenagers
    climbing accidents, 93
    flash flood victims, 11, 13–14, 15, 24,
        26–32
    hiking and falls over cliffs, 58–61,
        69–71, 72–73, 78
    hiking and hyperthermia, 162–63
    slickrock falls over cliffs, 73–74
Teichner, Don, 38, 40, 44
Temple of Aeolus. See Angels Landing
Temple of Sinawava, 2, 13, 26, 96
tents, 142–43

Terry, Ron, 18, 21, 59
Terry, Tommy, 15
Tersigni, Rob, 60, 62–63, 142, 143
Thanksgiving hikes, 84–86
Thompson, Ron, 33
thunderstorms, 170
timber industry and equipment, 151–53,
    156–57
Toler, Sarah, 142–43
Toogood, Theron, 73, 74
Touchstone, 102–3
Towers of the Virgin, 46
trail registries, 166
trails. See also hiking; specific names of trails
    to Angels Landing, descriptions, 49–51
    danger descriptions, overview, 72
    easy, 2
    flash floods impacting, 45–47
    Hop Valley, descriptions, 162
    safety precautions, 68, 71–72
    safety tips for children on, 45
    vehicular accidents on firefighting,
        145–46
Tuell, Shawn, 84
tunnels. See Zion-Mt. Carmel Tunnel, The
Tuttle, Matt, 102

Upper Emerald Pool and waterfall, 76
US Geological Survey, 9
Utah Canyoneering Guide (website), 50
Utah National Parks Council, 61
Utah State University faculty members,
    84–86

Valencia Hiking Crew, 38–45
Vander Meer, Bernadette, 62
Vander Meer, David, 62–63
Van Leuven, Chris, 114, 115
vehicular accidents
    common causes of, 145
    driving and safety guidelines, 165
    on firefighting trail, 145–46
    motorcycles, 126–28, 129–30, 144–45
    rollovers, 146–48
Vint, Thomas Chalmers, 49
Virgin River. See Narrows of the Virgin
    River
visitor roles and responsibilities. See also
    safety guidelines

personal culpability, 36–37, 71–72, 89
personal limitation acknowledgment,
    50, 168
situational awareness, 109
Vo, Douglas Yoshi, 21–23

Wa, Yi Jien, 80
walking sticks, 2
Walter's Wiggles, 49–50
Washington County Water Conservancy
    District (WCD), 33, 35–37
waterfalls
    climbing accidents, 93
    falls off edges, 79
    inexperienced canyoneers and
        rappelling accidents, 105–8
    rainstorms creating, 45–46
    safety guidelines for, 172
    slickrock and falls off, 76
    slickrock stream falls over, 86–88
water-related accidents. *See* floods, flash
water safety, 170–72
water supplies, 167, 169, 171
water treatment tools, 167–68
weather conditions. *See also* floods, flash;
        storms
    airplane crashes, 148–50
    flash flood indicators, 170–71
    unpredictability of, 45, 47
Webb, Kenneth, 14–15, 15
Weeping Rock trailhead, 83
Welling, Angie, 140–41
Welton, James Martin, 102–3
Westover, John H., 127
West Rim Trail, 49, 58
West Temple, 46, 78, 119–20
Whitworth, Jock, 107, 109
Widow's Tree, 50
wildlife, 172–74
Winder, Ether, 153–56
Winder, John, 155
wingsuit jumping, 118
Woolsey, Brad, 149–50
Wright, Kurt, 7, 17

Yengich, Ronald, 139, 140
Yosemite National Park, 37, 172

Zion Adventure Company, 19–20, 38
Zion Lodge
    drinking water access, 169
    employees, 72, 79
    missing visitors, 57–58
    vehicular accidents and nursing
        facilities at, 144
Zion-Mt. Carmel Tunnel, The
    bicycle rider accidents, 128, 130–31
    construction accidents at, 124–25
    descriptions, 122
    design and construction, 122–23
    lawsuits on design negligence, 126–28
    lost balance over rock wall deaths at,
        125
    motorcycle accidents and deaths,
        126–28, 129–30
    oversized vehicle usage policies,
        128–29
    traffic through, 125–26
    usage restrictions (bicycles,
        pedestrians), 129
Zion National Park
    annual death statistics, iv
    commercial guides, restrictions on, 39
    death statistics, 164
    emergency medical service (EMS)
        calls, statistics, 110, 111
    history, iv
    residential history, 151
    safety information and warnings, 8–9,
        37, 45
    timber industry history, 151–53,
        156–57
    visitor statistics, 108
    website for, 8–9
    websites about, 2, 46, 70, 132–33
    wrongful death lawsuits, 33–34
Zion National Park (Taylor), 152
ZionNational-Park.com, 46, 70
Zion Park Inn employees, 73

ABOUT THE AUTHOR

Randi Minetor has written more than forty books for Globe Pequot, including *Zion and Bryce Canyon National Parks Pocket Guide*, *Death in Glacier National Park*, *Historic Glacier National Park*, *Backyard Birding*, *Hiking Waterfalls in New York*, *Scenic Routes & Byways New York*, *Day Trips Hudson Valley*, and *Hiking Through History New York*. She lives in Rochester, New York.